PSYCHOVENEREOLOGY

Sexual Medicine, Volume 3
HAROLD I. LIEF, M.D., SERIES EDITOR

OTHER VOLUMES IN THE SERIES

PSYCHOVENEREOLOGY

Personality and Lifestyle Factors in Sexually Transmitted Diseases in Homosexual Men

Michael W. Ross

PRAEGER

New York
Westport, Connecticut
London

Library of Congress Cataloging in Publication Data

Ross, Michael W., 1952-
  Psychovenereology : personality and lifestyle factors
in sexually transmitted diseases in homosexual men.

  (Sexual medicine series ; v. 3)
  Bibliography: p.
  Includes index.
  1. Venereal diseases — Psychological aspects.
2. Homosexuals — Diseases — Psychological aspects.
3. Homosexuals, Male — Psychology.   I. Title.
II. Series [DNLM: 1. Homosexuality.   2. Men —
psychology.   3. Venereal Diseases — psychology.
W1 SE99F v.3 / WC 140 R825p]
RC200.1.R67   1986   616.95′1′0019   85-25683
ISBN 0-275-92122-0 (alk. paper)

Library of Congress Catalog Card Number: 85-25683
ISBN: 0-275-92122-0

First published in 1986

Praeger Publishers, 521 Fifth Avenue, New York, NY 10175
A division of Greenwood Press, Inc.

Printed in the United States of America

The paper used in this book complies with the Permanent
Paper Standard issued by the National Information Standards
Organization (Z39.48-1984).

10 9 8 7 6 5 4 3 2 1

To Peter, whose support and understanding made the completion of this book possible.

Foreword

Psychovenereology is a new concept. It deals with the social and psychological dimensions of behavior that are etiologically significant in the acquisition of sexually transmitted diseases, and with the same dimensions of the behavior of people who have become infected. There is a new branch of inquiry that is helpful to epidemiologists, basic scientists, clinicians, and social scientists. The material in this book should help all those who wish to deepen their understanding of the interaction of the many variables that lead to and flow from the acquisitions of STDs.

AIDS is an epidemic that has frightened the world. What do we know about the behaviors that play such an important role in contracting AIDS? What do we know about the behavior of patients with AIDS, especially their sexual behavior? What do we know about ways in which through better understanding we may modify the spread of the disease?

Mike Ross applies sophisticated research methods to his investigation of these and related questions. He has chosen homosexual men for his investigation (although he plans to use similar methods in a forthcoming investigation of heterosexuals), men because gay women have a very low incidence of STDs and homosexual men because of the relatively high frequency of STDs among them, because the stigma attached to homosexual behavior intensifies and magnifies psychological factors, and because homosexual research respondents tend to be disproportionately well educated and cooperative to researchers.

This brief foreword can hardly do justice to the broad scope of this volume. For example, a separate chapter is devoted to "illness, behavior, and STD infection" dealing with how infection modifies the sexual behavior and lifestyles of those infected, and another chapter is devoted to "psychoimmunology and homosexual men." Since the lymphocytic system (of which the "T" helper cells are part) is such an integral aspect of the immune system, and since it is the latter that is damaged or destroyed in AIDS, the role of stress in affecting the immune system and the impact of the damaged immune system on the brain (and on behavior) are current "hot topics" of investigation.

Mike Ross is to be commended for the groundbreaking work, and I am delighted to add it to our series on "Sexual Medicine." His is the third volume in the Series to be published.

Harold I. Lief, M.D.

Preface

The initial stimulus for my interest in the psychosocial bases of sexually transmitted diseases in homosexual men came when, as a graduate student in New Zealand in the mid-1970s, I was introduced to the argument that higher rates of STDs in gay men justified the criminalization of homosexual behavior. This lead to reading in the area and to the production of my paper on homosexuality and venereal disease in the *British Journal of Sexual Medicine* in 1979. In that first attempt to spell out what I believed were the social, psychological, and political contributors to an increased incidence of STDs in some groups of gay men, it became clear that there were a number of hypotheses of major interest that had not received any adequate formulation and testing. I subsequently included questions on venereal diseases in my major four-country study of homosexuality and was able to test, discard, and modify many of my implicit hypotheses, some of which were correct, some incorrect, and many overly simplistic.

However, since the news of AIDS had begun to impinge on medical, if not public, consciousness in 1981, the issue of homosexuality and STDs had taken on a new importance. Now the issue had an applied relevance it lacked when STD infections were seen as of little more significance than the common cold, and recognition of this stimulated me to prepare some of my data for publication. Coincidentally, at a meeting in Philadelphia with Dr. Harold Lief of the University of Pennsylvania Medical School in which we discussed our common interest in sexual education in medical school curricula, he suggested that the area of psycho-venereology might make a useful monograph in the series he was editing. This in turn led to further data collection and reorganization of my thoughts in the area, and to present the work.

At the time of writing this, AIDS has become a major public health hazard in the gay community and beyond, and variables which may affect its transmission have not only academic interest but may be vital in decreasing the spread of the virus and in reducing mortality. For this reason, the work reported here is important not only in terms of

providing some baselines that will help us to understand,
and thus help, individuals who wish to modify sexual behaviors that increase risk, but also in terms of its generation of additional hypotheses and research studies.
Hopefully, this work will have a more general impact as
well, in that it will legitimize the area of psychovenereology
as a valid and important topic of study in its own right,
with heterosexual and homosexual, male and female samples.

Having made the point of the applied importance of
psychovenereology at this point in the development of the
AIDS epidemic, I should also point out my implicit assumptions about the interface of psychology, sociology, and
venereology. I do not believe that homosexual behavior is
intrinsically different from heterosexual behavior. Nor do I
believe that homosexual individuals are intrinsically different from heterosexual individuals except, in Western
societies, in the nature and strength of stigma directed
toward them. One may identify sexual behaviors, regardless of the genders of the participants, that carry a
greater risk of STD transmission than others, and such
behaviors need to be modified if the risks of infection in
terms of morbidity or mortality outweigh the pleasures of
these particular behaviors. In the case of AIDS, the risks
are major, and hence this work is on homosexual men rather
than heterosexual men or women or homosexual women. I
do hope, however, to follow this volume with work on the
psychovenereology of heterosexual men, since there is no
reason why many of the principles that appear to underlie
sexual behavior in homosexual men should not apply equally
to heterosexual men.

Lest this study be interpreted as another attempt to
medicalize homosexuality, I should also like to make it clear
that I do not see enforced modification of at-risk behaviors
in homosexual men as either possible or ethical. It is a
fact of life that AIDS, as a medical disorder, has to date
struck disproportionate numbers of homosexual men, and
that this has of necessity medicalized homosexual health
care and aspects of homosexual behavior. Hopefully, at
some time in the future if a vaccine becomes feasible, the
area will become demedicalized to a significant degree.
However, it may also be argued that attempting to modify
some homosexual sexual behaviors is tantamount to a devaluation of homosexuality. I do not agree: what is argued in
this work is that some forms of homosexual behavior are
less risky than others, and that if individuals wish to lower
risk, then a shift to alternative homosexual practices may
be appropriate. Given the highly cathected nature of
sexual behavior, it is almost impossible to modify it on one's

own, and for this reason an understanding of the forces that impel people in the direction of particular sexual behaviors is critical. We know only too well from the literature on modification of other potential health risks such as smoking and dietary concommitants of coronary artery disease that information on its own will modify the at-risk behaviors of less than 10 percent of individuals. With such a heavily psychologically invested area as sexual behavior, individuals are most probably going to need much greater insight into and understanding of their sexual needs to modify particular preferences. The data contained in this work will, hopefully, go some way to assisting this.

While I have argued that homosexual behavior is an intrinsically rewarding and as intrinsically natural as heterosexual behavior, I have also noted areas where some homosexual behaviors are driven by factors that could be associated both with healthy acceptance of one's sexuality and with less mature approaches to sexual expression. I am keenly aware that many of my findings and arguments will be able to be taken out of context and used as justification for devaluing homosexuals (despite the fact that they may apply equally well to heterosexuals), or for the purposes of justifying homosexuality. However, I believe that the existence of bigotry or homophobia is no justification for the suppression of scientific discussion, particularly when the price paid for avoiding the topic may now be measured in human lives.

This book has the unenviable aim of serving two masters: the medical and scientific research community by providing basic data and discussion on the psychological and social concommitants of STDs in homosexual men, and those in applied areas of public health who have the responsibility of helping homosexual men individually and collectively to reduce the risk of contracting AIDS and other STDs. Whether I have come near to achieving either of these two aims remains to be seen, but if I have succeeded in making psychovenereology a valid discipline for research and discussion, and in providing some information that may assist in understanding and modifying risk factors for STD infection and our treatment of individuals with STDs, then I will have more than achieved my objectives.

Acknowledgements

My greatest debt, as in all my research into homosexual populations, is to all those who are the source of the information contained within this book, but who must remain nameless. A debt of almost the same magnitude is due to those organizations that gave me access to their mailing list, including Society Five and the Metropolitan Community Church in Melbourne, Camp Inc. and the Metropolitan Community Church in Brisbane, RFSL in Stockholm, SETA in Helsinki, and the National Gay Federation in Dublin. The four-country study was itself part of a larger study and was only made possible by two generous travel grants from the Faculty of Arts of the University of Melbourne. My thanks also go to the gay community in Adelaide and to the South Australian Health Commission who funded Dr. Paul Drew and myself to commence a study on the homosexual population in South Australia.

The environment in which research is carried out is no less critical than the research content, and my thanks go to Professor Ross Kalucy and Associate Professor Julian Hafner of the Department of Psychiatry, the Flinders University Medical School, Adelaide, for providing a stimulating and accepting environment for what must have seemed a very unusual research area. An equal debt of thanks goes to my colleagues on the National Venereology Council of Australia, Dr. Ross Philpot, Dr. David Bradford, Dr. Marten Lindon, and Dr. Jillian Need, and Dr. Paul Drew of the University of Adelaide Medical School, who have consistently supported and encouraged what from their perspective must have seemed a strange juxtaposition of clinical areas. Similarly, the social and political implications of my work, especially in the environment of AIDS, must be acknowledged, and I have to thank my friends and colleagues Dr. Jim Paulsen of Stanford University Medical School and Dr. David Ostrow of Northwestern University Medical School for helping me to see beyond my data. A generous travel grant from the Michael Q. Petersen Memorial Fund enabled me to deliver the first memorial lecture to the American Physicians for Human Rights in Chicago in 1984 and without this Chapter 4, on which the lecture was based, would not have been written.

The collection of the California data reported in Chapter 9 would not have been possible without the generous help of Dr. Richard Hamilton and Dr. William Owens, and they have my thanks for this. I also appreciate the help of Dr. Kevin White of Flinders University in pointing out some of the sociological literature in the area of venereology, and Peter Saunders, Flinders University Medical Librarian, for his compilation of the index.

Any authors will know that good secretaries are worth more than their weight in gold, and the superb contribution of Janine Judd, who managed the manuscript with her usual cheerful efficiency despite the arrival of Benjamin, has my thanks and admiration. Finally, the example provided by the pioneers in this area, Dr. William Darrow and Dr. Gavin Hart, must be acknowledged in the contributions their writings made to the development of my ideas and of this book. However, despite the great moral and intellectual debts I owe to my friends and colleagues, any errors in this work will be mine and I take full responsibility for them.

Contents

Appendixes

About the Author

This is what I gathered.
That in that country if a man
falls into ill-health, or catches any
disorder, or fails bodily in any way . . .
he is tried before a jury of his
countrymen, and if convicted is held up
to public scorn and sentenced more
or less severely as the case may be.

Samuel Butler
Erewhon

1

Introduction to Psychovenereology

In 1973, Hart stated that sexually related diseases are "a behavioural problem, the control of which requires focus on the fundamental personality of the individual." Over the past decade, research has implicated to a greater and greater extent that social and psychological variables as well as frank psychodiagnostic issues are intimately involved in transmission of sexually related diseases. A systematic attempt to describe these variables is long overdue, and the discipline of psychovenereology has begun to emerge in response to the need for models to quantify the relationships between psyche and pathogen.

Psychovenereology is an area of investigation that describes the interaction of two sets of factors in human disease: psychological factors such as personality and lifestyle, and their relationship to rates of contraction of sexually related diseases. When a sexually related disease is contracted, psychovenereology also describes the associated illness behaviors (which are quite different from those in socially accepted disorders) and the subsequent reactions to the sexually related disease that incorporate the meaning of the disease to the individual and may determine subsequent behavior and compliance with treatment.

Transmission of a sexually related disease requires much more than the juxtaposition of secretion or mucous membrane with receptive surface or blood. There is a chain of events that leads up to the transmission of a pathogen, including sexual behaviors that provide the

1

necessary contact, behaviors which take the individual to geographical location where risk may be higher in terms of prevalence of pathogens, and the factors that lead to increase of risk through increased partner numbers. These, however, are only the more direct determinants.

Less direct determinants of whether an individual contracts a sexually related disease will include not only the psychological states which may underlie partner numbers, indulgence in particular sexual practices, and frequenting high-risk locales but such variables as pre- and postsexual precautions against infection, knowledge about sexually related diseases to ensure their recognition, frequency of checks if high-risk behavior is common, and reactions to disease and subsequent attendance for treatment and compliance with treatment. There is a psychological basis for all these behaviors that will affect everything related to treatment from an initial attendance through to contact-tracing. Given that many individuals will be asymptomatic carriers or may not notice or recognize early symptoms until several further sexual contacts have been made, the importance of psychological factors cannot be overestimated. In fact, this book provides data that consistently suggest that psychosocial variables are the *best* predictors of who will contract a sexually related disease, and that understanding of such diseases and preventative measures must concentrate on psychological aspects of venereology.

It is possible, however, to go even beyond these risk-related factors in psychovenereology. It has been recognized for some time that psychological factors may predetermine the presentation of many disease states ranging from coronary heart disease (the predisposer being the so-called "Type A" personality (Jenkins, Rosenman and Friedman 1967) to acute appendicitis (where loss and socially undesirable or uncontrollable events in the past three months may best account for the 72 percent of histologically normal appendixes removed from young girls (Canton, Santonastaso and Fraccon 1984). With sexually related diseases, the strongly cathected nature of all sexual activity probably acts as a multiplier for such conventional precursors, along with the lack of reliable information about sexuality, the taboos surrounding it, and the lack of discussion of sexual matters in Western societies.

The term psychovenereology, as a consequence, also covers the pathological reactions to sexually related diseases and in fact to sexuality itself. Hart (1977) has previously used the term *venereoneurosis* to describe the symptoms that characterize the significant number of individuals who present and re-present to venereal disease clinics without any evidence of disease but frequently with marked evidence of sexually related guilt or more severe psychopathology. Even in those with demonstrable infection, Catalan et al. (1981) have demonstrated that some 40 percent of clinic attenders are psychiatric cases using a conventional screening test, and some 25 percent of males and 40 percent of females had a sexual dysfunction. Clearly, the psychological component of clinic attendance is in itself sufficient to warrant special consideration in any coverage of psychovenereology. With sexual minorities such as homosexual men, of course, there are added components of major complexity and concern such as stages of "coming out," internalized homophobia, and a degree of social stigma that further enhances the importance of psychological factors in the practice of venereology.

The most recent, and perhaps the most medically exciting, aspect of psychovenereology does involve what occurs when pathogenic organisms invade the body. At this point, the body's immune system becomes involved and there are a number of links between the immune system and psychological states. As far back as 1978, Ader demonstrated that the immune system in laboratory animals could be classically conditioned, thus demonstrating clear links between psychological states and immune function, which has lead to the rapid recent development of psychoneuroimmunology (Ader 1981). Initially, it was recognized that acute stress had the effect of raising cortisol levels, which in turn depressed immune function, but more recently it has become clear that the relationship is by no means as simple and that numerous aspects of lifestyle both in the distant past as well as immediate can cause immunodepression or enhancement. Blalock (1984) has gone so far as to suggest that the immune system acts as a sensory organ in that it is a bidirectional system: the nervous system may affect lymphocytes and lymphocyte changes may affect the nervous system, acting as an integrated circuit.

In the light of experimental evidence to date, then, psychovenereology is in a position to provide some clarification to questions as to why some individuals develop infections when exposed to a pathogen, others develop subclinical infection or become carriers, and yet others develop antibodies without any evidence of illness. While there are clearly a large number of variables involved as currently demonstrated by the evidence to date on hepatitis B and acquired immune deficiency syndrome (AIDS), there appears to be sufficient evidence to implicate psychological factors as one of the cofactors involved. Thus psychovenereology addresses a whole chain of events ranging from high-risk behaviors and their psychological determinants to some of the direct determinants of infection and the psychological consequences of infection.

This book concentrates on the homosexual man in the study of psychovenereology. The reasons for this are both coincidental and deliberate. The coincidental reasons relate to the particular interest in homosexual men with the advent of AIDS and the clinical and preventative importance of understanding some of the variables that may affect at-risk behaviors, transmission, and infection. The deliberate reasons for concentrating on homosexual men are multiple.

Perhaps the most important is the relative frequency of sexually related diseases in some subsections of the homosexual population. Ross (1984a) found that between 32 and 48 percent of homosexual men sampled in four countries had had a sexually related disease, and Darrow et al. (1981) found a similar figure of 78 percent for the United States. Both of these studies were derived from research that was looking at questions unrelated to sexually transmitted disease in homosexual populations: on the other hand, because a random sample of homosexuals is impossible to obtain, most samples overrepresent the more sexually and socially active.

Of equal importance is the fact that in most Western societies, homosexuality is stigmatized. In looking at the psychological precursors and sequelae of sexually related diseases, this stigma will have the effect of intensifying psychological factors and magnifying them. There are, of course, inherent dangers in using homosexual men as a model, though, as Ostrow (1984) has pointed out: it is very easy to imply that there is some psychopathology in homosexuality by concentrating on such a group, despite the fact that it is abundantly clear that homosexuality is a normal variant of sexual behavior and as such unrelated to any psychopathology. In this book, it is implicitly assumed that there is no essential psychological difference between homosexual and heterosexual behaviors, and that homosexual and heterosexual interactions (both emotional and physical) may have positive or negative connotations depending on context and motivations. Any problems associated with a male homosexual lifestyle are likely to be a function of societal pressures (Ross 1985e) and not evidence of psychopathology. In contrast, not only do homosexual women have a lower incidence of sexually related diseases than heterosexual women (Robertson and Schacter 1981) but they also appear to display superior psychological functioning to heterosexual women (Freedman 1971): for these reasons, they are perhaps the most inappropriate group in which to

research psychovenereology. Ostrow also notes that unless
we describe side by side the various typologies of sexual
behavior, and not just those found in STD clinic attenders,
we are in danger of remedicalizing the 1950s view that
infection and psychopathology are linked. For this reason,
studies of STD clinic attenders without comparable control
groups are likely to be both dangerous and misleading.

The third reason that homosexual men are an excellent
group in which to study psychovenereology is that, in
contrast to heterosexual men with a high incidence of
sexually related diseases, homosexual respondents in research tend to be disproportionately well educated and
cooperative to researchers. As a result of these differences between homosexual and heterosexual men with high
incidences of sexually related diseases, by using homosexual
respondents it is possible to lessen the influence of
confounders such as socioeconomic class as well as to obtain
accurate responses. Nevertheless, the advantage of having
a relatively high incidence of sexually related diseases
without any confounders such as psychopathology or variation in socioeconomic status, coupled with the presence of
stigmatized sexual orientation, makes homosexual men an
appropriate group for investigation. The need to understand the environment in which a significant proportion of
AIDS cases occur underscores the appropriateness of this
group.

Psychovenereology as an area of investigation, however,
covers all sectors of the sexually active population. It is
an amalgam of the disciplines of epidemiology, social and
preventative medicine, psychosomatic medicine, psychiatry,
and immunology applied to the content area of sexually
related disease. This book explores these areas and dem-
onstrates that a substantial proportion of the variance of
incidence of sexually related diseases can be accounted for
by psychological factors that lead to at-risk sexual practices and lifestyles, immunodepression, lack of concern
about symptoms and compliance with treatment, and abnormal illness behavior, and describes the dimensions of attitudes to sexual behavior in homosexual men.

By the end of this book, the importance of the data
presented here for the understanding and appropriate
treatment of patients with sexually related diseases should
be apparent, as should the importance of establishing
educative and preventative measures where the patterns of
infection-related behavior may be broken. Ultimately, we
have to recognize that any area of medicine so intimately
connected with sexuality will contain a complex interrela-
tionship of highly cathected forces that demonstrate the

accuracy of the comment by Darrow (1981) that venereal disease is not so much a medical problem with some behavioral aspects as it is a social problem with some medical aspects.

2

Social and Psychological Aspects of Sexually Transmitted Diseases: The Research Background

Previous research on social and psychological aspects of STDs has been infrequently carried out, and where it has been done, has frequently made use of biased samples. Nevertheless, there are a number of common findings across researchers that provide an outline of social and psychological factors that influence the rate of contraction of STDs. One of the most common findings is the higher incidence of STDs in homosexual men as compared to heterosexual men (Ostrow and Altman 1983), and a lower incidence of STDs in homosexual women as compared to heterosexual women (Robertson and Schacter 1981). The wide discrepancies between these four groups underscores the fact that a homosexual orientation, whether in males or females, is not the causal factor: neither is gender by itself a cause. It could be postulated, however, that a gender-related variable may be linked with higher incidence of STDs. If a male-associated variable predisposes to infection, then a male-male relationship would be expected to provide the highest incidence of STD infection, and a female-female relationship the lowest, as is the case. Alternatively, anatomical variables could be postulated, such as the relative protection offered by the cornified epithelium of the vagina as opposed to the squamous epithelium of the rectum. This, however, raises a second issue of the different sexual behaviors associated with male-male, female-male and female-female behaviors as an important factor in STD transmission.

Ostrow and Altman (1983), reviewing the literature on homosexual lifestyles and STDs, report that across studies there is general agreement that homosexual men have a significantly higher incidence of STDs, including syphilis, gonorrhea, viral hepatitis, nongonococcal (nonspecific) urethritis, proctitis, herpes simplex type II (herpes genitalis), amebiasis, giardiasis, shigellosis, and anal warts. To this list Handsfield (1981) has added hepatitis A and hepatitis non-A non-B, enteritis due to *Campylobacter fetus,* genital and meningicoccal infections, and cytomegalovirus. On the other hand, Stamm et al. (1984) report a higher incidence of urethral *Chlamydia trachomatis* in heterosexual men than in homosexual men, and Fulford et al. (1983a) noted that hepatitis and syphilis rates were highest in homosexual men, non-specific urethritis highest in heterosexual men, and gonorrhea highest in bisexual men. Nevertheless, from the best evidence to hand, the Gay Report on STDs of Darrow et al. (1981), in order of frequency of those who had never had the following STDs came *Pediculosis pubis* (31.9 percent), gonorrhea (60 percent), non-specific urethritis (72.7 percent), genital warts (79.6 percent), scabies (80.7 percent), syphilis (85.2 percent), genital herpes (87.1 percent), and hepatitis B (87.7 percent): however, only 30 percent were not seropositive for antigen or antibody to hepatitis B. Of all Darrow et al.'s sample, only 22 percent had never had an STD; if *Pediculosis pubis* is excluded, the figure is 40 percent. Similarly, Ross (1984) found that in the four countries he studied, the percentage never infected with an STD ranged from 52.3 percent (Sweden) to 68 percent (Ireland). There seems little doubt that homosexual men do account for a disproportionate amount of STD infection, at least in the Western world. However, it is of interest to note that Fluker (1983) has pointed out that this phenomenon has occurred only since World War II.

It must be recognized, however, that what data we have to generalize from are in all cases subject to bias. Ostrow and Altman (1983) note that most if not all studies they report on were conducted in STD clinics, and this leads to bias toward public clinic attenders, as well as a lack of control groups. There are probably only two adequate studies that allow us to look at incidence, those of Darrow et al. (1981) and Ross (1984a). The study of Darrow et al. contains one of the largest samples of homosexual men ever investigated (4,212), and was derived from a study into numerous other variables as well as STDs. It has nevertheless been criticized by Handsfield (1981) for having a response rate of only 1.5 percent. The

study by Ross (1984a), while on a much smaller sample of
604 respondents, had response rates of between 44 percent
and 54 percent and was carried out in four different countries, thus giving an opportunity for independent replicates. This study was also part of an investigation into
variables other than STDs. Both studies had the major
advantage of being carried out in the community and not in
an STD clinic as well as having controls from the same
sources. They further point out the bias of researching
groups from public STD clinics, since in Darrow et al.'s
study only 42.7 percent attended gay or public clinics,
while the proportions attending public clinics in Ross's
study ranged from 80.2 percent (Sweden) to 40 percent
(Australia). These figures point to the danger of generalizing from public clinic groups, which according to
Darrow et al. tend to be younger, and more unhappy with
their treatment. Those who wanted to keep their sexual
orientation secret tended to go to private practitioners, and
an astonishing number (from 20.5 percent in Sweden to 52.3
percent in Finland) did not admit the source of their infection to be homosexual.

Practitioner attitudes have been heavily implicated in
failure to disclose sexual orientation. Pauly and Goldstein
(1970) reported that 75 percent of a sample of 1,000 medical
practitioners admitted they felt uncomfortable with homosexual patients, while Sandholzer (1980) reports more
recently that one-third of physicians were sometimes or
often uncomfortable with homosexual patients and 84 percent
felt that homosexual patients hesitated to seek help because
of physician disapproval. Not surprisingly, Dardick and
Grady (1980) indicate that some 49 percent of homosexual
men don't tell their primary medical practitioner of their
sexual orientation. Ross (1984a) notes that between 13.7
percent and 18.2 percent of respondents in his four-country study had had negative experiences in public STD
clinics, and Ross and Stalstrom (1984) found in Finland that
these were almost entirely negative attitudes on the part of
the physician. In an earlier study on attitudes to STD
clinics in Australian homosexual men, Ross (1981) also
found physician attitudes, and to a less extent clinic environment and perceived level of hygiene, leading to dissatisfaction. As a consequence, great caution must be taken
in looking at characteristics of homosexual men who attend
either public clinics or private physicians, since there are
likely to be major biases both from choice of venue for
medical care and from level of admission of a homosexual
lifestyle.

Before discussing in detail the social and psychological

factors that are associated with STD infection in homosexual men, it is appropriate to briefly review the factors that are associated with STD infection in homosexuals. One of the best reviews in the literature on environmental and individual factors influencing STD infection is provided by Hart (1977). He notes that the sexual behavior of the individual may change suddenly and dramatically in response to personal or environmental stress, and illustrates this by way of his own thorough and perceptive studies of sexual behavior and venereal disease in a war environment (Hart 1973a,b, 1974, 1975). Environmental stresses Hart includes in addition to a war environment include separation from the stable community on which the individual has relied for social expression, for example, a travel-related profession, institutionalization, or social turmoil or migration. Superimposed on major environmental stresses may be lesser stressors such as loneliness, conflict with superiors or peers, low job satisfaction, or difficulties with interpersonal relationships. It is particularly interesting in the context of this book to note that these lesser stressors may all lead to loss of self-esteem.

Other individual factors that Hart (1977) notes may be associated with an increase in risk for STDs include the following variables:

- *Race:* black Americans have a higher infection rate than white Americans, as do Maoris compared to whites in New Zealand and Aboriginals compared to whites in Australia. These differences are probably due to a higher rate of intercourse and with higher-risk partners in the nonwhite populations.
- *Age:* high infection rates tend to occur in younger groups, since this is the more sexually active group of the population. Most venereal disease occurs in the under 30 age group. However, a number of studies have failed to show a relationship between age and infection.
- *Marital Status:* STDs are normally less common among the married population, although individuals who are divorced, separated, or widowed may be at greater risk than single persons. Marital discord or breakdown is likely to lead to atypical sexual behavior and subsequent infection.
- *Education:* there tends to be an inverse relationship between STDs and education, with the better educated having fewer infections (the most dramatic reduction occurring in the tertiary educated group). It is doubtful, however, if intelligence has any relationship to

STD infection.
- *Socioeconomic Status:* many studies have suggested an inverse relationship between STD infection and socioeconomic status, but this latter variable is difficult to define. It may be that better educated and higher socioeconomic status individuals are less likely to attend public clinics and thus are disproportionately represented in the statistics.
- *Parental Influence:* parental discord or marital disruption is a common feature in the background of individuals with STD infection. Those infected are likely to come from larger families (usually more than four children) and to have had a stricter upbringing.
- *Associated Crime:* there is a consistent relationship between criminal offenses and venereal infection, and both are, according to Hart, manifestations of underlying social maladjustment. However, both could also be reflections of underlying dimensions of sex-role-related acting out or reactions to stressors.
- *Attitudes and Beliefs:* there has not been any consistent relationship reported between knowledge of STDs and infection, but physician attitudes may have a bearing on patient's attitudes and presentation for treatment. While strength of religious belief has been inversely associated with STD infection, this is not a consistent finding in recent studies.
- *Alcohol:* the association between alcohol and STD infection is a strong one. It is uncertain, however, whether alcohol disinhibits individuals who then enter into casual unions, whether alcohol is the excuse for STD infections, or whether high-risk encounters mostly occur in bars and clubs where alcohol is also available. Hart also notes that there is probably an underlying personality dimension which predisposes to both drinking and high-risk behavior for STD infection; that is, numerous sexual encounters, often with prostitutes. A relationship between alcohol abuse and gonorrhea in homosexual men was also found by Fulford et al. (1983b).
- *Personal Prophylaxis:* those individuals who use a condom may be at lower risk than nonusers, although Hart suggests that condoms probably have an insignificant effect in controlling STD infection, as does washing the genitals or flushing the urethra following intercourse.

In terms of personality variables relating to a higher incidence of STD infection in heterosexuals, Hart notes that extraversion is a powerful prediction, and that sociopathic personality or personality disorder may cause promiscuity. He goes so far as to suggest that the relationships of the social factors outlined above may be secondary to STD infection, with attitudinal and personality variables being primary causes of increased STD infection. If this is the case, we would expect the social and demographic variables to be unrelated to STD infection in homosexuals, and attitudinal and personality variables to be consistent across sexual orientation. It is therefore appropriate at this point to review the social, and psychological, concommitants of STD infections in homosexual men.

Ostrow and Altman (1983) suggest that there are four areas of interest to investigate if the question of why homosexual men have a higher incidence of STDs is to be satisfactorily answered. These areas include behaviors (sexual practices, partner numbers, and anonymity of contacts); cultural variables such as the attitude of health-care providers, the public, and patients themselves to homosexuality; legal and political variables; and physical factors such as the virulence and pathogenic nature of the STD agents and physical features that may mask signs and symptoms. To this list can also be added two further variables, demographic variables and psychological variables. These areas will be dealt with in turn.

DEMOGRAPHIC FACTORS

Several demographic factors can be identified as being related to incidence of STD infection in homosexual men. Ostrow and Altman noted that the number of years an individual had been homosexually active was a good indicator of the number of STDs contracted: similarly, Darrow et al. (1981) found that the time individuals had been homosexually active was a good predictor of number of infections, along with age. Age is probably a mechanistic variable, allowing for more opportunity to contract an STD, all other factors being equal. There are consistent findings from the work of Hooker (1964) that the highest age group for STD infection in homosexual men was 20–24, similar to the at-risk group in heterosexuals. Darrow et al. also noted that a second good predictor was whether individuals came from a larger metropolitan area, as opposed to smaller towns or rural areas. Similarly, Fluker (1981) reported that there was wide variation in the number of cases of homosexually acquired syphilis in the London metropolitan area, and almost none in rural areas. Figures coming from public clinics in London show an interesting geographical bias. Estimates range from as high as 84 percent of presenting cases of early syphilis in London homosexually acquired (Waugh 1972) to a mere 6 percent (Oriel 1971). Such a vast range in the same city at the same time illustrates geographical bias *within* a city. Wilcox (1973) also reports that there is an almost linear relationship between the size of a city and the proportion of homosexually acquired STDs. In London, specifically in three hospitals in the West End, 27.9 percent of the national total of primary and secondary syphilis, and 9.8 percent of gonorrhea, were treated. This reflects the movement of some homosexuals to large centers of population, but it is also apparent that attitudes at particular clinics have a major effect. Wilcox notes that at nearly a quarter of the London clinics 80 percent of the STDs were homosexually acquired. Such clinics encouraged homosexuals to attend, and this explains the discrepancy in statistics within London. Significantly, Thin and Smith (1976) noted that the boroughs with the highest proportion of individuals presenting with homosexually acquired STDs were quite distant from the West London clinics: apparently, individuals will travel some distance to an accepting clinic.

This evidence suggests that homosexuals tend to congregate in metropolitan centers, and possibly that those who are interested in large numbers of partners tend to move to cities to facilitate their lifestyle. Interestingly, Hooker has also reported that compared with heterosexuals, far more homosexual men with syphilis are both employed and better educated. In view of the differences within the United Kingdom for figures for homosexually acquired syphilis (Wales, 9.5 percent; Scotland, 13.5 percent; England, 46 percent) given by Wilcox (1973), it is clear that demographic factors have a major influence on patterns of STD infection.

SEXUAL PRACTICES

While there has always been a recognition that sexual practices are likely to be intimately involved with STD infection (and hence the terms venereal disease and sexually transmissible disease), it is often difficult to go beyond this truism. Clearly, an activity such as mutual masturbation is unlikely to result in the spread of pathogens, but since many sexual encounters consist of numerous sexual activities, it is difficult to tease out any interrelationships between specific acts and infection. Nevertheless, some consistent findings to date have been reported, particularly for hepatitis B.

Schreeder et al. (1982) noted that anal intercourse and analingus were both major risk factors for transmission of hepatitis B, and Darrow et al. (1981) also note these activities as risk factors for gonorrhea. Similarly, an oral-anal route has been implicated for hepatitis A in homosexual men by Christenson et al. (1982). Ross (1985a) reported that for syphilis and gonorrhea, an oral sex preference was a predictor of low levels of infection, while anal intercourse and other anal practices such as brachioproctic erotic activity (" fist-fucking ") were predictors of high infection rates. Fulford et al. (1983c) also found anal passivity significantly correlated with syphilis, although negatively with gonorrhea and nonspecific urethritis. More recently, research into risk factors for AIDS has implicated passive anal intercourse and active analingus.

Specific sexual practices have also been implicated in an apparent overrepresentation of presumed homosexual men with cancer of the anus or rectum (Daling et al. 1982) and more specifically squamous cell carcinoma (Austin 1982). It has been suggested that passive anal intercourse leads to fissures and tears as well as perirectal abscesses and nonspecific proctitis (McMillan and Lee 1981). As well as being implicated in transmission of hepatitis B, AIDS, gonorrhea, and possibly rectal cancer, passive anal intercourse is probably implicated in the spread of infection since anal or rectal symptoms are likely to go unnoticed more frequently than genital or oral ones. As an example, Ostrow and Altman note that between 21 and 68 percent of gonorrhea in homosexual men is asymptomatic: even mild symptoms are likely to go unnoticed if they are anorectal.

However, despite the fact that some authors such as Fulford et al. (1983c) believe sexual activity to be equally important as promiscuity in determining STD risk, it may not be specific sexual practices themselves that act as direct predictors of infection, but the fact that some particular practices are associated with either high partner numbers or preference for particular locations for sexual encounters. For example, individuals who make sexual contact in public toilets are far more likely to indulge in oral sex or mutual masturbation (Humphreys 1970), and brachioproctic practices more likely to occur in back-room bars or steam baths specifically catering to those interested in sadomasochistic activities. On the other hand, specific activities such as active analingus are far more likely to lead to transmission of enteric parasites than any other sexual practice. It is therefore important to determine whether it is the sexual practices themselves or their association with other at-risk activities such as high partner numbers or sexual contact at particular locales that are associated with higher rates of STD infection. While Judson (1977) has argued that "if we are to reduce the incidence of sexually transmitted diseases, we must encourage some basic changes in sexual behaviour," we must first establish precisely which sexual behaviors are at greatest risk for each disease, and which are at least risk, before proceeding to argue for alterations in specific sexual practices.

PARTNER NUMBERS

Numbers of sexual partners have long been recognized as one of the major risk factors for STD infection. Numerous researchers have noted that number of partners is one of the better predictors of infection (Ostrow and Altman 1983, Darrow et al. 1981) although Darrow et al. found that number of lifetime partners was a significant correlate for syphilis and hepatitis B but not for gonorrhea. More than 50 different lifetime sexual partners significantly increased the possibility of herpes, hepatitis B and syphilis. Schreeder et al. (1982), however, make a distinction between steady and nonsteady partners, and found the latter a predictor of hepatitis B infection.

On the other hand, Hooker (1964) reports that promiscuity appeared unrelated to syphilis infection in a study carried out in Los Angeles in 1961. Other more recent studies (Fulford et al. 1983c) have reported that bisexual men have higher partner numbers than homosexual men, who in turn have higher numbers than heterosexual men. But several researchers, including Henderson (1977) have suggested that multiple partners are not so important as the *type* of partner in the sexual contact. In this context it is interesting that Ross (1984b) found that partner numbers were not a significant predictor of STD infection in Sweden, Finland, and Australia (but were in Ireland) using a multiple regression design. It may be, then, that partner numbers are a significant variable only in the context of sexual practices, partner characteristics, and the pathogen involved. Ross (1982) found partner numbers related to transmission of infection only in diseases with a long latency period, since this allowed more partners to become infected prior to the appearance of symptoms and treatment. The most frequently reported partner characteristic in the literature is anonymity of sexual contact.

PARTNER CHARACTERISTICS

Henderson (1977) has argued that anonymity of partner is one of the most important contributors to STD infection because it does not allow for interruption of the chain of transmission. Data available have suggested that "furtive activities" are significant risk factors for syphilis, hepatitis B, and other STDs, but not gonorrhea. Darrow et al. (1981) report that as the frequency of sexual activity in gay baths, parks and bushes, public toilets, bars and peep shows and pornographic movie houses decreased so did self-reports of hepatitis. This association was in fact significant regardless of age, number of partners, or size of place of residence. It has been suggested (Ross 1984c) that the importance of partner anonymity lies in the fact that places where partners are anonymous are also places where multiple partners may be contacted: the association with two partners who have each had eight partners increases the risk factor by 16. Certainly casual partners, who are often also anonymous, have been implicated in STD infection levels by Fulford et al. (1983c) for both homosexual and heterosexual men. However, Oriel (1982) has argued that such variables as compulsive promiscuity are in fact due to emotional insecurity or personality disorders. It is therefore of central importance to examine the evidence for psychological factors as the underlying dimension in partner numbers, sexual practices, and partner anonymity.

PSYCHOLOGICAL VARIABLES

Hart (1973b) has argued not only that there is "increasing recognition of venereal disease as a behavioral disease," but also that all the sociological variables implicated in venereal disease are primarily related to the personality of the individual. He reported for his heterosexual sample that an increase in extraversion, and to a lesser extent neuroticism as measured by the Eysenck Personality Inventory, were associated with increased STD infection and appeared to underly many of the sociological variables he found to differentiate his infected and noninfected groups. Similar peaks on neuroticism for both heterosexual and homosexual men were noted by Wells and Schofield (1972), although they found their homosexual patients to be more introverted than the heterosexuals, and by Fulford et al. (1983b) who found significant and positive correlations between neuroticism and syphilis and gonorrhea infection in their total homosexual and heterosexual sample. They also reported that clinic patients scored higher on psychoticism, extra-version, and neuroticism when compared with Eysenck's norms, and that bisexuals had the highest elevations of neuroticism and psychoticism compared to homosexual and heterosexual men. Measured on Eysenck's Sexual Attitudes Inventory, Fulford et al. found clinic subjects generally to be less interested than Eysenck's controls in physical sex and pornography, to have less sexual excitement, and greater prudishness, sexual disgust, and neurotic sexual attitudes. Homosexual patients did not differ from heterosexual patients, but surprisingly the bisexual patients accounted for most of these differences between clinic patients and controls. They also found bisexual men to be the only group with evidence of psychological disorder.

While there is some evidence of increased scores on personality traits such as neuroticism and extraversion for those individuals with STD infections, most studies took patients presenting at STD clinics and failed to discriminate between those with a single infection and those with multiple infections. Further difficulties in interpretation arise from use of test norms as control groups without establishing the degree of comparability. Although some studies have established that some 40 percent of heterosexual patients at STD clinics are likely psychiatric cases based on screening questionnaires (Catalan et al. 1981), Pedder and Goldberg 1970), there has been little evidence of actual disorder but considerable speculation about the possible underlying psychodynamics of individuals who contract STDs.

In 1964, Hooker suggested that the homosexual man who "seeks escape from loneliness and guilt in 'compulsive cruising' . . . is more likely to be infected with an STD." Oriel (1982) has also suggested that compulsive promiscuity is due to emotional insecurity or personality disorders. Parental relationships have also been suggested as a contributing factor in STD infections. Morton (1966) saw the "lack of an intelligent and affectionate approach by parents" as a causative factor, and Fluker (1983) writes of unhappy homes, parental indifference, overcrowding, and parental severity as further contributors. It is of particular interest that Hart (1973a) has reported that soldiers coming from large (four or more children) families as being significantly more at risk for STD infection, and Ross (1984b,c) reports that parental relationships are among the significant predictors of multiple STD infections in the four countries he studied.

Other psychological factors may have both direct and indirect effects on infection rates, particularly environmental stresses. Hart (1973a) has noted in his classic studies of STDs in troops in Vietnam that "the environmental stresses of war produced behaviour patterns which many would not otherwise experience." The stresses of immigration are similarly acknowledged by Armytage (1980) who comments that half of the men with gonorrhea in the United Kingdom in the 1960s were immigrants, and Oriel (1982) also notes that single migrants frequently have numerous sexual encounters until they settle into their new cultural background. This apparently holds for nonwestern societies, as Hart (1974) has reported that in single laborers and married immigrants in Papua New Guinea, recourse to prostitutes and, to a lesser extent, homosexual behavior, are more common outlets and venereal disease is a prominent sequel. There is some very convincing evidence in the numerous studies in which STD incidence rates in immigrants and soldiers are increased markedly (in comparison to baseline rates prior to immigration or war) that instability and insecurity resulting from a change to an alien culture or environment is associated with lack of discrimination in, or increase in frequency of, sexual contacts.

It could be argued that in most Western societies, a homosexual orientation is one which both produces stress and removes individuals from the seemingly stable and secure heterosexual culture they have been brought up in: they thus become "sexual immigrants" within their own society. The association of stress with STD infection as a test of this hypothesis would provide some indication of whether the stress of a homosexual orientation is a contributor to the increased incidence of STDs in homosexual men.

On the other hand, a little-cited but important study by Kelus (1973) in Poland took random samples of STD clinic attenders and inhabitants in a town near Warsaw and found no differences between inhabitants and patients apart from a tendency for patients to be more urbanized and less religious. However, Kelus provided two models to describe how neuroticism or psychological problems might lead to different sequelae in terms of STDs, which can be schematically represented:

| Neuroticism | Promiscuity | STDs |
| Neuroticism | Sexual Inhibition | STDs |

While this model sees the influence on STD incidence as occurring through partner numbers alone, it does implicate self-esteem as an intervening variable preceding partner numbers. Perhaps more importantly, Kelus suggests that in more permissive societies, neuroticism would lead to *prom-iscuity,* while in the more restrictive society, neuroticism would lead to *sexual inhibition.* Thus, how the individual copes with his psyche in relation to his sexuality depends on the cultural context of that individual. It is of interest that Ross (1984a) found that there was a lower level of STDs in homosexual men in the two smallest and most agrarian countries studied, Finland and Ireland, and the highest in the two largest and most industrialized and cosmopolitan societies, Sweden and Australia, providing indirect support for the hypothesis put forward by Kelus. The emphasis placed by Kelus on cultural background does suggest, however, that cultural factors may influence STD incidence rates.

On the other hand, Hooker (1964) has suggested that "for some, the seeking of sexual contacts with other males is an activity which is isolated from all other aspects of their lives." We cannot assume that psychological factors that influence partner contacts will be obvious in other areas of the individual's life, but perhaps only in specifically sexual attitudes.

CULTURAL VARIABLES

Included among cultural variables are political and legal stances on homosexuality that vary from society to society, since these may affect both sexual behavior and admission of the source of infection. While Fluker (1983) has noted that the incidence of STD infection in homosexual men has increased since World War II, there is no certainty as to why this has occurred. Ostrow and Altman (1983) have canvased a number of possibilities: the influence of the Gay Liberation movements in the late 1960s and early 1970s, the increase in homosexual steam baths and saunas and the possibility of anonymous contacts, and the increasing variation in sexual practices as a result of the so-called sexual revolution that followed from such phenomena as the Kinsey reports, the advent of the anovulent pill, and the protest movements of the late 1960s. While the effects of these occurrences are probably interwoven, the net result was to allow homosexuality to become more open and to allow more overt concentrations of homosexuals to develop.

Without doubt, there has been a change in the homosexual lifestyle, which has been well documented and which has heralded a within-culture alteration of attitudes toward sexual variations. Hooker's research on homosexual men in 1961 (Hooker 1964) lead her to remark that "the 'one-night stand' is the standard expectation and monogamous fidelity rare." Gebhard and Johnson (1979), reporting on Kinsey's homosexual data (collected between 1938 and 1963) gave a median value of 20 for number of lifetime partners. Bell and Weinberg (1978) however, in a sample collected in 1970 in the San Francisco Bay area, report that 60 percent of their white male respondents had over 250 lifetime contacts, compared with 44 percent of their black male respondents, in fact, more than half of the black men, and white men had had more than 20 partners in the preceding year. Bell and Weinberg's sample is probably biased in favor of those with high partner numbers by its geographical location in one of the more homosexual cities in the world, since Darrow et al. found the median number of sexual partners in a lifetime in the San Francisco respondents in their sample to be 200. Nevertheless, it would still appear that there has been a radical increase in partner numbers over time. With such an increase, the increase in the incidence of homosexually acquired STDs comes as no surprise: however, it is also apparent that there are substantial subcultural variations within homosexuals, and patterns of at-risk behaviors and disease probably differ in the large metropolitan areas compared to the rest of the country.

A further consideration already alluded to earlier that may have some effect on STD incidence relates to diagnostic issues. The World Health Organization (1975) noted that where homosexual activity is illegal or heavily stigmatized, the source of infection will probably not be reported as homosexual. This may have the effect of preempting investigation of rectal or oral sites by the physician, and coupled with the previously noted inability of many physicians to cope with homosexual patients and the reluctance of homosexual patients to reveal their sexual orientation to their physicians, may lead to underreporting and inappropriate investigation. The World Health Organization also notes the tendency for homosexual men to congregate in metropolitan areas to safeguard their anonymity, and to form closed circles where STDs spread rapidly, where homosexuality is stigmatized or illegal. The effect of law changes in this regard is amply demonstrated by Suhonen et al. (1976). They reported the incidence of primary syphilis increasing from 8 percent prior to decriminalization of homosexual acts in Finland in 1970 to 50 percent in 1974–1975. That the percentage of individuals reporting homosexually transmitted syphilis rose *without* the total numbers increasing significantly indicates that decriminalization has no effect on the incidence of STDs, but only on accuracy of reporting.

Political and legal status of homosexuality clearly has an influence on reporting, since stigma will have the effect of discouraging honesty and encouraging anonymous contacts. There are, however, other cultural variables that may affect both incidence and pattern of STDs in particular societies. Ross (1984a) has suggested that there are likely to be more STD infections and reinfections in the industrialized nations he studied (Sweden and Australia) and less in the agrarian ones (Finland and Ireland). The Swedish figures in fact are comparable to the rates of infection found by Darrow et al. for the United States in the same year. Cultural factors of this nature occur also in research on heterosexually acquired STDs: Arya and Bennett (1967) found that in East Africa the traditional inverse relationship found between social class and gonorrhea infection was reversed, with gonorrhea being a major health problem in the elite group in the universities.

However, in comparing the patterns of STD infection in homosexual men both with heterosexual men and with homosexual men in different cultures, one must be aware that there may be few commonalities. Indeed, Hart (1973a) has proposed that there is a tendency to generalize about venereal disease by building a composite picture from participants in widely differing environments. While he was referring to patterns of STD infections in soldiers in a war environment as opposed to peace, and overseas as opposed to at home, his argument is a pertinent one. We have seen that almost none of the variables which are associated with STDs in heterosexual men are associated with STDs in homosexual men, and that different patterns of infection may occur in homosexual men in major metropolitan areas compared with smaller towns, and in different cultures. If there are any common elements, they should be able to be identified across cultures, and at the same time culture-bound elements may also be identified.

Nevertheless, the comment of Hart (1973b) that venereal disease is increasingly being recognized as a behavioral disease appears to accurately reflect the evidence summarized in this chapter. Essentially, the evidence for common social factors affecting STD incidence in both homosexual and heterosexual men is weak, and the little evidence for psychological factors suggests that personality and psychological factors may explain more of the variance in STDs than social or physical variables.

It could be argued that the determinants of most sexual behavior are sexual attitudes, and that the reason there is little common pattern between homosexual and heterosexual men in terms of STD precursors is that sexual attitudes and beliefs about the purpose and meaning of sexuality are different. It is therefore probable that family background, personality, self-perceptions, and sexual attitudes together will account for a substantial proportion of the variance in partner numbers, sexual practices, anonymity of partner, and partner preference, all of which have been implicated in levels of STDs. Nevertheless, it must also be accepted that there is an element of chance in STD infection and that a complete explanation of its precursors and concommitants is impossible. However, any understanding of the etiology of STDs makes explanation and intervention possible, and it is by following the pointers provided by the background literature that empirical investigation should commence.

3

Background, Samples, and Methods

This book reports on several studies, which are grouped together to allow both cross-cultural perspectives on psychosocial correlates of STDs in homosexual men, and replications of findings to establish consistency. Replication also serves the function of providing an opportunity to test additional hypotheses generated by the first studies. In one sense, all the studies reported here are an attempt to generate some basic data on psychovenereology in homosexual men and to allow for very specific hypotheses to be set up and tested. What follows is a description of the four societies in which the data were collected (Sweden, Finland, Ireland, and Australia) with, in Australia, separate descriptions of the two states included in the first study (Queensland and Victoria) and the state in which the second study was conducted (South Australia). Following on from these sketches of the legal and social status of homosexuality in these countries and states are the descriptions of the samples.

SWEDEN

Homosexuality in Sweden was dealt with only in the Lutheran Church law until 1864, in which the offense of "unzucht" (crime against nature) applied to sexual acts with a person of the same sex, male or female. While this law was removed from the statute books in 1944, higher age limits were retained with the heterosexual age of consent 15, homosexual 18. The 1944 change followed a campaign in the parliament since 1931, in which the Social Democrat member of parliament Wilhelm Lundstedt, who had had a married homosexual brother who had been blackmailed and suicided, had encouraged law reform, with little opposition.

Following the 1944 law change, there were two public scandals which brought the issue of homosexuality into the public arena. The first, the Haijby scandal, involved blackmail of the court of King Gustav V Adolf, with whom Haijby had fairly intimate connections. Haijby was subsequently charged with and punished for blackmail after the King's death in 1950.

The second scandal, the Kejne scandal, involved a Lutheran priest who was engaged in social work in slums. Some of his workmates sexually abused some boys, and although Kejne complained, no action was taken. He then claimed a "homosexual conspiracy," and began a campaign to "save Sweden from the homosexual conspiracy." The publicity grew immense, and led to public hysteria and witch-hunts in high places and by the police. The result was a parliamentary commission that took place over a period of two to three years, and found nothing. Kejne then accused the commission of being homosexual, which led to a second commission! As a result of the Kejne scandal, the 1950s were regarded as a decade of terror by homosexuals, with police harassment, blackmailings, and suicides.

It was against this background that RFSL (Riksforbundet for Sexeullt Likaberattigande) was founded in 1950, as a local chapter of the Danish 1948 Society. The organization began in an attempt to provide contact between homosexuals, social evenings, and to fight against the laws which discriminated against homosexuals. Social work in the homosexual community was emphasized, and the importance of having meeting places in the larger towns led to the 1950s also being known as the "decade of dance evenings."

Political action commenced with a letter to one of the liberal political parties in 1954 regarding the age of consent for homosexual acts, and contact with the Ministry of Justice. Local chapters of RFSL formed in other areas of the country apart from Stockholm, and four or five openly homosexual individuals began approaching political parties and publicizing the issue in the press and on the radio. By the end of the 1950s, a pen-pal chapter had been formed, and information services and leaflets to schools and to the authorities were being provided. By 1957, there were two chapters in Stockholm (male and female), and in

1964 they bought the Timmy Club through a major fund-raising effort.

In 1970, there was a major change: the Stonewall movement and Gay Liberation were making their mark in the United States, and younger people became involved as a result of such inspiration. While this lead to a degree of conflict in which younger and more radical individuals gained control of RFSL, there was a concerted effort to build up more local chapters, smaller groups, and actively to encourage openness. There was active dialogue with the authorities and discussion in schools, and RFSL became well-known. By 1973 there had been a considerable degree of lobbying of the parliament, which subsequently agreed that homosexuals living together were acceptable from the point of view of society. In 1977 there was a parliamentary commission on which all five parties were represented to investigate the conditions of homosexuals in Sweden, and in 1978 the age limit was lowered to 15, in line with the heterosexual age of consent. Homosexuals were able to join the military forces and the police without discrimination. The first results of the parliamentary commission were published in 1981 as a discussion paper on matrimony for homosexuals, and legal solutions to the issue. Some recommendations suggested by organizations who responded to the discussion paper included recognition of homosexual relationships as de facto unions, registration of such unions for the purposes of inheritance and other legal matters, and accepting homosexual unions as a state of matrimony. There was also some dissent, notably from the fundamentalist and pentecostal churches who recommended "readjustment centres!"

At the same time, RFSL had been steadily expanding, with 15 local chapters (all with premises), social evenings and dances at Club Timmy, and since May 1979 a twice-weekly Gay Radio program on Sundays and Thursdays for an hour each. The government sponsors some of these activities. Speakers to schools are provided by five local chapters (with problems arising from a lack of sufficient homosexual speakers, not schools), a telephone counseling service in Stockholm, Uppsala, and Goteborg has been set up, and a central social and political group has formed.

Sex education in Swedish schools with regard to homosexuality entered a new phase with the introduction of a new text in 1975, the chapter on homosexuality being written by RFSL. RFSL also produces a magazine, *Kom Ut* (Come Out) regularly in which there is debate on topics of interest to the homosexual community. Psychiatric attitudes have also come into line with public attitudes, with the classification of homosexuality as a disorder (World Health Organization category 302.00) being removed in Sweden in 1979 by the Ministry of Health.

Recent trends include the opening of a Gay bookshop in 1981, and openness about homosexuality becoming much more widespread. RFSL had a large membership (1,600 in 1980) of which about 30 percent are women, with some chapters, such as Malmo, having a preponderance of women. The openness of parliament and governmental and educational authorities in Sweden to consider the issue of homosexuality rationally has characterized the legal and social attitudes to homosexuals, and enormously aided the efforts of the homosexual community itself to gain acceptance and integration into society.

FINLAND

In Finland, the first criminalization of homosexual behavior was recorded in the twelfth century, under the laws of the Swedish crown, in which the penalty was a small fine. This remained the case until in 1628 the laws of Brandenburg-Prussia were imposed, which introduced the penalty of burning at the stake for homosexual acts. This penalty for "unnatural acts" was repeated in the Finnish Constitution of 1734, under Swedish occupation, and the Swedish laws applied while Finland was a Russian Grand Duchy from 1809 to 1917. Since that date, it has been an independent state. There was no change to the law from 1886, when homosexuality was first mentioned and two years imprisonment the penalty, until 1971, when homosexuality was decriminalized. Under the 1971 law, the age of consent for homosexual acts was set at 18 (21 if one partner is in a position of authority), and the corresponding ages for heterosexual acts were 16 (18). Penalities also differ, with prison being mandatory for homosexual offenses, but not for heterosexual ones. However, these laws at present are not commonly used, and in practice are "dead laws."

At the time of the decriminalization of 1971, however, the law RL20:9:2 was enacted as a trade-off with the state (Lutheran) church for decriminalization. This law provided for a fine or six months imprisonment as penalty for any positive publicity about homosexuality, on the assumption that this would "propagate" homosexuality (Ross and Talikka 1978). This law, far from being a dead law, has been used in two censorship cases since 1971. In 1976, the Finnish Broadcasting Corporation was prosecuted for showing a film on the founder of the Metropolitan Community

Church in the United States, and for announcing the decision of the American Psychiatric Association to remove homosexuality as such from its classification of mental disorders. Both cases were referred to the Public Prosecutor, and in both cases the charges were dropped as there was insufficient evidence or the court decided there was no case to answer. However, the threat of prosecution is still an important determinant of what newspapers and the broadcasting commission publish or broadcast. There has, however, since 1978, been some positive reporting of homosexuality without prosecution, although the law still stands.

Unfortunately, the negative information on homosexuality extends to medical texts, with all current Finnish psychiatric texts basing their views of homosexuality on the psychoanalytic opinions of Allen and Bieber and his colleagues, which suggests that homosexuality is a mental disorder in which individuals in behavior and personality resemble the opposite sex and that other perversions and psychoses are associated with homosexuality. Homosexuals, these texts report, form subcultures and are incapable of human relationships. Most studies reported are of patients, prisoners, or rats. A similar approach is taken in the main textbook of clinical psychology. Thus official texts see homosexuals as lonely, depressed, and suffering people who spread their disease by seduction.

With such official attitudes and despite law changes, it is perhaps surprising that decriminalization occurred in 1971. The liberal attitudes of the late 1960s and the report of the nonparliamentary law reform committee of 1966 provided the impetus for a private member's bill to be introduced by the (conservative) parliamentary opposition which was subsequently passed. There has subsequently been a private members' bill introduced in 1977 attempting to remove the law RL20:9:2, but no action has been taken on this. The suggestion that the laws for homosexual and heterosexual acts be equalized has similarly not been acted on.

Social organization of homosexuals in Finland sprang from the so-called "November Movement" of 1966, which was generally liberal and anti-authoritarian, and which had a homosexual section. From this, in 1969, Psyke, a homosexual organization, was founded composed mainly of males with goals of decriminalization of homosexual acts, social acceptance, and provision of social outlets and a club for homosexuals. It also published, with an emphasis on soft pornography and love stories. In May 1974 a splinter group in Psyke that was opposed to the semi-pornography published and that wanted public action was formed, calling

itself SETA (Seksuaalinen Tasavertaisuus ry: Organisation
for Sexual Equality). Composed initially of males, it became
jointly male and female after a year, and since 1974 has
been publicly active. It has sought newspaper publicity
and made formal statements about the position of homosexuals and need for law reform to the Ministries of Justice, Health and Social Affairs. It instigated the private
member's bill introduced to repeal the censorship law, has
lobbied extensively members of parliament, and holds peri-
odic demonstrations. Seminars and lectures to groups are
delivered, and more recently television programs have been
prepared and screened. Community services are also
emphasized, with a Gay Switchboard, commencing in 1974,
running for three days a week from 18:00 to 21:00 hours
and having training sessions with mental health professionals. Socially, SETA also runs a disco two evenings a week
and has an office and drop-in, along with introductory
coffee evenings. Subgroups include a women's group,
Christian group, communist group and a music group, as
well as the research arm of the movement. Since 1975, a
magazine (including an English edition) has been published
bimonthly, since 1979 with a state grant in assistance, and
is used as a part of university courses and includes papers
by academics.

Membership is skewed toward younger members, with
many students, and in 1981 was about 1,300, with a male:fe-
male ratio of about 7:3. At present, SETA is heavily
involved in public education and attempts to alter those
remaining laws that discriminate against homosexuality.
Public education is regarded as particularly important since
the sex education books (about 20 different ones) used in
schools for 16- to 18-year-olds repeat the attitudes of
psychiatric and psychological texts that homosexuality is a
mental disorder and leads to guilt, loneliness, and failure.
There is thus a contradiction in Finland between legal
status and the attitudes of some professions to the issue.

AUSTRALIA

Data in Australia were taken from three of the eight states
and territories, Queensland (northeast), Victoria (south-
east), and South Australia (south central). At the time of
data collection (early 1978), neither Victoria nor Queensland
had reformed its laws with regard to homosexual behavior
between males, but Victoria subsequently did so three years
later, in 1981. South Australia has had a remarkably
liberal set of laws in place since 1975, and data (for the

second study) were collected in 1984. Since there are between-state differences, the three states are dealt with separately.

Victoria

The legal status of homosexuality at the time of the present research, in both Victoria and Queensland, was based on the English Offences Against the Person Act of 1861, in which buggery was subject to life imprisonment or up to ten years imprisonment if attempted, and the Criminal Law Amendment Act of 1885 in which indecent behavior between males was subject to a penalty of up to two years imprisonment. These laws were subsequently modified to remove minimum penalties, but remained in force although were not widely enforced. Prior to 1861, the 1533 Statute of Henry VIII punishing buggery with death or lesser punishment would have been the appropriate statute.

Attempts in Victoria to amend these laws commenced in early 1976, when a homosexual electoral lobby was formed prior to a state election, and this became the Homosexual Law Reform Coalition (HLRC) a couple of months later. The HLRC was an umbrella group representing the homosexual organizations of Victoria, and commenced to coordinate attempts at law reform. In 1974, the opposition (Labor) party had supported homosexual law reform in caucus, and this was subsequently supported at the party's state conference in 1975. A private member's bill was introduced by a Labor member at the end of 1975, but was not debated. The HLRC had meetings with the member who introduced the bill in 1976, and an amended bill was introduced in 1977; this bill was never voted on. The government, the Liberal (conservative) party, had supported homosexual law reform in 1974, and the Young Liberal Movement had also urged some moves to be made in late 1976 at their annual conference. In March of 1977 the Liberal premier of Victoria agreed to act on this policy, and persuaded his government to support such a change to the law. Impetus may have been provided by a national homosexual conference in Melbourne, the capital of Victoria, in 1979 to proceed with the bill, but this is not clear. At the time of obtaining the Victorian sample (March-April 1978), homosexual behavior between males was criminalized (although rarely if ever enforced), and some attempts at law reform had been made, with both major political parties supporting such a move in principle.

Subsequently, a bill which removed the criminal classification of homosexuality and made it the equal of heterosexuality (the law applied usually to homosexuals and heterosexuals with regard to age of consent and indecency) was introduced as a government measure in late 1980, passed and proclaimed law in 1981.

Social organizations in Victoria were not founded formally until 1971, when Society 5 was formed as a group to provide social and political support for male homosexuals. At about the same time, the more radical Gay Liberation Front (GLF) was formed at the University of Melbourne in 1972, and provided both support for students and dances at the university. Society 5 had its own premises, which were open in the evenings and included a dance floor, telephone counseling service, library and speakers to outside organizations. While GLF included women, Society 5 did not. Prior to the advent of these two groups, most homosexual social contact took place in a few selected hotel bars in Melbourne.

In the mid-1970s, other groups such as the Gay Teachers and Students Group, the Australian Gay Archives, and the Metropolitan Community Church (which started in Melbourne in 1974 and attracted a substantial homosexual congregation) existed, the latter two in a loose association with GLF. From 1976 a Gay Radio Collective was formed, and broadcast for an hour once-weekly on a commercial station. The HLRC became an umbrella body with links and representatives from all these bodies, although Society 5 (and more recently, the Metropolitan Community Church) remained the only bodies with premises. Socially, the majority of homosexual men still met in selected hotel bars, and there was no organized group apart from Society 5 and the loosely organized GLF.

Publicity about homosexuality was sparse until late 1976, when police at Black Rock, a southern Melbourne beachside suburb, began a campaign against homosexuals who tended to use the beach and the adjacent shrubbery for cruising. Homosexuals appeared for the first time on television to protest this harassment, and publicity in the major metropolitan newspaper occurred which was fair and supportive of law reform. While there had been occasional publicity since the introduction of the first private member's bill in 1975, it had been intermittent and not particularly visible.

Further publicity came about in 1979, where two males were arrested for kissing outside a gay bar in Melbourne, charged with offensive behavior in a public place, and fined. This lead to a major "kiss-in" (at which no arrests were made!) by some members of the homosexual community in late 1979 as further publicity for the need for law reform. Since 1979, there has also been a magazine produced by the HLRC, whereas previously only the Society 5 newsletter had been a regular publication, although restricted to members.

At the time of data collection, male homosexuals in Victoria were strongly discriminated against in law, although this law was rarely enforced and there was evidence that law reform was being considered.

Queensland

As in Victoria, the law in Queensland is based on the Labouchere amendment of 1885 which, with minor modifications, is in force at the present. Unlike Victoria, there have been no attempts to change the law, and none of the political parties in Queensland have homosexual law reform as part of their platform.

The only major homosexual organization, CAMP Inc., was founded in 1972 and has its own clubrooms, and phone line ("phone-a-friend") for information and counseling. There has been a small congregation of the Metropolitan Community Church in Brisbane since 1974, and since the data were collected in 1978, there have been a number of gay groups formed, including a university group, a Gay Radio Media group that broadcasts for an hour weekly, and more recently Gay Action Alliance, a more radical group than CAMP. CAMP (an acronym standing for Campaign Against Moral Persecution) was founded in order to provide a focus for homosexual social activity at about the time that Society 5 was founded in Victoria, when homosexual issues were beginning to be aired publicly following the Stonewall Riots in New York in 1969 and the formation of the Gay Liberation Front in the United States. In Queensland, however, publicity has not been either common or positive, and CAMP has concentrated on serving the homosexual community.

Public reaction to homosexuality, if the governmental reaction is any indication, is extremely negative, and police regularly harass known homosexual cruising places and arrests are frequent. It is rare, however, for imprisonment to result and arrests are usually on the basis of gross indecency rather than for specifically homosexual acts. The police also raided and forced to close a predominantly homosexual sauna establishment in 1980. In general, Queensland has the same legal basis as Victoria for criminalization of homosexuals, but laws are enforced and both governmental and, presumably, public attitudes toward homosexuality are much more negative. As a result homosexual groups are much more inward-looking and reticent about publicity, and there is some danger of prosecutions for homosexual behavior if it is associated with cruising.

South Australia

As in the other Australian states, the law in South Australia was based on English statutes of the Offences Against the Person Act of 1861 and the Criminal Law Amendment Act of 1885. In 1971, a branch of Campaign Against Moral Persecution (CAMP) was founded in South Australia, a few months after it was founded in Sydney, New South Wales. This organization was founded like so many others in the activist climate that followed the Stonewall Riots and the formation of Gay Liberation groups in the United States. About the same time, the first exclusively homosexual club, the AC/DC Club, was opened in Adelaide, the state capital.

The stimulus for law reform was the drowning of Dr. George Duncan, a Professor of Law at the University of Adelaide, in May 1972. Dr. Duncan was thrown into the River Torrens in Adelaide next to a popular cruising area by three men. Three members of the police vice squad were dismissed after they had refused to answer questions put to them by a superior officer relating to the possibility of their presence near, or involvement in, the murder (Parkin 1981). Several months later a member of the State Upper House, the Legislative Council, introduced a bill to decriminalize homosexual acts between consenting males. This bill, amended to make it a defense that homosexual acts were between consenting adults in private, passed, although the age of consent for homosexuals was 21, and 16 for heterosexuals. In 1973 the Labour Attorney General, Peter Duncan, introduced a bill in the Lower House to totally amend the legislation relating to sexual offenses by removing any reference to gender of partner so that there was complete equality between homosexuals and heterosexuals. This bill passed the Lower House but was defeated in the Upper House on the casting vote of the President of the Legislative Council, following some damaging and ill-timed publicity over teaching about homosexuality in schools by the newly formed Gay Activists Alliance. Following a state election that changed the composition of the Upper House, the same bill was introduced by Peter Duncan and passed both houses in 1975. From this time, all sexual offenses applied equally to homosexuals and heterosexuals, and homosexuals thus had complete equality in law in matters such as age of consent, sexual assault, and indecency provisions.

During the period between the murder of Dr. Duncan and the successful bill sponsored by Peter Duncan, a number of homosexual groups had been founded, including the Metropolitan Community Church, and a bookshop, the Dr. Duncan Revolution Bookshop (1974–1978). From 1976, further organization occurred in the gay community, including the opening of a gay sauna, a social club (1346 Club) that held annual Gay Olympics, a motorcycle club, a men's center that became the nucleus of the Gay Counselling Service in 1976, and from 1978 to 1980 the Adelaide Homosexual Alliance, which formed to protest at police action against homosexual cruising areas in Adelaide. University Gay Societies were founded at the two universities, the University of Adelaide (1972) and Flinders University (1978), which still continue to operate, and both organized dances and social events. Since the passing of the Duncan Bill in 1975, a number of gay bars and discos have opened in Adelaide.

In 1984, the Labour Government introduced as government policy a bill to outlaw discrimination on a number of grounds, including homosexuality, which was passed and became law in the same year. As a result, South Australia has removed legal discrimination against homosexuals and indeed made it illegal to discriminate, as well as being the first Australian state to decriminalize homosexual behavior. Also in 1984, with the first cases of AIDS being reported in Australia (although none in South Australia), the AIDS Action Committee was set up as an umbrella group to coordinate information and action to prevent the spread of AIDS.

REPUBLIC OF IRELAND

It is not surprising that the Republic of Ireland (Eire), having been a part of the United Kingdom and under the British crown from the Norman invasion of 1169 to independence in 1922, was subject to British law. Subsequent to the 1533 act of Henry VIII of England already referred to, an act of the Irish parliament of 1634 introduced the buggery provisions into Irish law, and provided that those convicted should suffer death as a felon. With the passing of the Offences Against the Person Act of 1861, the penalty became penal servitude for life or a minimum of ten years, although with the enactment of Section 2 of the Penal Servitude Act of 1891, courts could impose at their discretion imprisonment of two years. The British laws of 1861 and 1885 applied in Ireland as they did in Australia, and on independence in 1922, were incorporated into Irish law unchanged, still as Sections 61 and 62 of the Offences Against the Person Act (1861) and Section 11 of the Criminal Law (Amendment) Act of 1885 (the latter the infamous Labouchere amendment). This 1885 act was the law under which the famous Irish aesthete Oscar Wilde was imprisoned in 1895, and which was unsuccessfully challenged in the case of Norris versus Attorney-General in 1977.

There was little organized homosexual activity of a social or political nature in Ireland (apart from one or two predominantly homosexual hotel bars in Dublin) until a conference on human sexuality was held at the New University of Ulster at Coleraine, from which emerged a steering committee charged with the creation of a union for sexual freedom in Ireland. Within the universities in Derry, Coleraine, Belfast, and Dublin, branches of the Sexual Liberation Movement arose. A symposium on homosexuality at Trinity College, Dublin, led to the formation of the Irish Gay Rights Movement in 1974. In 1977 the Campaign for Homosexual Law Reform was founded following the demise of the Irish Gay Rights Movement, and was followed in a short space of time by the Hirschfeld Foundation. By 1979, a building had been acquired and the National Gay Federation, an umbrella group of homosexual organizations, had been formed. It is uncertain whether there were any particular stimuli that produced an Irish homosexual movement in 1974, but in all probability it was founded as a politicization of homosexual issues and in line with the organization of homosexual movements that was taking place in Britain, Europe, and the United States in the early 1970s.

While the Irish Gay Rights Movement and National Gay Federation have publically called for homosexual law reform in the areas of criminal law, equal opportunities, taxation, and recognizing homosexual relationships, most notably in their first national conference in Cork in May 1981, there has been little public debate and no legislative action. One action in the courts (Norris versus Attorney General), while defeated on a technicality, did provide some publicity. At the time of data collection (early 1980), however, publicity had not been extensive.

Attitudes toward homosexuality in Ireland were measured by McGreil (1977), who found that in Dublin, 45.2 percent of adults believed that homosexual behavior between consenting adults should not be a crime. It is probable that by the time the sample was collected, this proportion may have reached 50 percent.

In Dublin, there are two associated movements, the National Gay Federation, and the Campaign for Homosexual Law Reform and the Hirschfeld Foundation, which have club rooms that include a cinema, discotheque, coffee bar, and telephone information and counseling service in their own respective buildings. Other services provided by this group include a youth group, befriending group, and a bimonthly publication, *In Touch,* an occasional publication, *Vortex,* as well as a monthly newsletter. While police appear to tacitly accept homosexuals and there have been no reports of consistent entrapment or harassment, the attitude of the Roman Catholic Church has been consistently negative, and the church has very considerable power in Ireland in terms of its power to both influence government and public opinion. As a result, homosexuality is viewed as a religious and moral sin rather than legal crime, and there is little hope of this view being modified. At the time of data collection, the homosexual movement in the Republic of Ireland was still concentrating on establishing itself within the homosexual community in Dublin, although the national conference in 1981, subsequent to data collection, saw a movement toward increasing publicity and pressure for government legislative reform. Until then, most publicity and action had been the work of one or two individuals.

In summary, the history and attitudes toward homosexuality and the legislation relating to homosexuals vary considerably between the four countries for which data are available. While it would be preferable to measure public attitudes, it is necessary to attempt to rank the four societies on the basis of their legislative and social responses to homosexuality. Clearly Sweden, with almost complete equality, ranks first, with Finland (legislative equality but not complete, and with some censorship) second. Australia is ranked third, with Victoria being antihomosexual in regard to legislation but clearly moving toward reform: Queensland is particularly antihomosexual with no prospect of law reform at the time of writing. Ireland is in much the same position as Queensland, although with less police activity and signs of more recent activity by homosexual groups. While there is not a great deal to separate these states, Australia is ranked third and Ireland fourth: despite the similarities between Queensland and Ireland, the situation in Victoria pulls Australia up slightly compared with Ireland. On the other hand, the situation in South Australia, source of the sample for the next study, more closely approximates that in Sweden.

It must be recognized, however, that such a ranking

system is crude and does little more than to indicate the aspects that homosexuals in each of these societies may note in attempting to assess the pro- or antihomosexual stance of their society. As such, it may give some indication, in conjunction with responses from homosexuals in these societies, of what variables are associated with attitudes to homosexuality in western Europe.

SUBJECTS AND METHODS, HOMOSEXUAL SAMPLES

Sample Population, Study One

The sample consisted of 176 Swedish, 158 Australian, 149 Finnish, and 121 Irish homosexual men (602 respondents in total). Characteristics of the sample are given in Table 3.1.

Samples were collected by giving questionnaires, complete with stamped addressed envelopes for return, to homosexual rights and social clubs in Stockholm, in Melbourne and Brisbane, in Helsinki, and in Dublin. In each of the cases the club was the main homosexual or social rights organization in that city, and the aims and functions of the five clubs selected appeared to be almost identical. The response rate was 46.4 percent for Stockholm, 44 percent for Melbourne and Brisbane, 54 percent for Helsinki, and 48.6 percent for Dublin. This rate was based on the number of questionnaires given to the clubs (equivalent to the number of men on their mailing lists).

Questionnaire

The questions asked were part of an anonymous wider questionnaire comparing homosexual men in Sweden, Australia, Finland, and Ireland. The questions asked appear in Appendix 1.

Instructions for the questionnaire were as follows:

> This questionnaire is part of a cross-cultural piece of research which is designed to examine the social and cultural factors which affect homosexuals in different societies which have different legal and social attitudes toward homosexuality. It consists of a series of questions and psychometric scales, particularly designed so that they can be compared statistically across societies. Some of these scales will have special instructions, which you should read carefully before commencing to score them. In

TABLE 3.1 Demographic Characteristics (Mean ± SD) of Samples of Homosexual Men in Four Countries

Variable	Sweden	Australia	Finland	Ireland	Differences
Age	30.9 ± 7.4	32.0 ± 11.4	28.4 ± 7.8	29.1 ± 9.7	Australia-Finland
Years of education	12.7 ± 5.3	13.3 ± 3.6	13.2 ± 4.4	13.5 ± 5.9	Ireland-Sweden*
Age at which became homosexually active	29.8 ± 7.4	19.3 ± 12.1	20.4 ± 7.2	20.9 ± 6.8	
Age realized was homosexual	14.1 ± 5.7	12.5 ± 7.0	13.9 ± 5.4	15.6 ± 6.0	
Kinsey scale level	6.6 ± 0.8	6.7 ± 1.0	6.5 ± 0.9	6.2 ± 1.0	
Sexual partners per month over past year	3.3 ± 6.2	2.7 ± 3.5	1.7 ± 2.6	2.0 ± 3.6	Sweden-Finland*
Religion (%)					
Practicing	11 (6.7)	52 (32.4)	10 (7.1)	37 (31.4)	
Nominal	91 (55.5)	51 (33.6)	66 (47.1)	48 (40.7)	$\chi^2_6 = 66.6$**
None	62 (37.8)	49 (32.2)	64 (45.7)	33 (28.0)	
Social class					
Upper	32 (18.9)	8 (5.2)	4 (2.8)	15 (12.4)	
Middle	80 (47.3)	89 (58.2)	66 (45.8)	72 (59.5)	$\chi^2_6 = 40.1$**
Working	57 (33.7)	56 (36.6)	74 (51.4)	34 (28.1)	

*$p < .05$.
**$p < .01$.

general, because this is a relatively long questionnaire, we suggest that the best idea is to put the
first response that comes into your head, and not
to think a long time about items: not only has it
been found that the first response is the most
accurate, but if you think too much about some of
the items, you may decide that it is impossible to
answer them accurately. If this happens, go back
and put your first general response to the question
as it applies to you. Almost all the questions
require only that you mark a scale or a box with [a
check] or [an x], or circle a letter (see sample
below). The questionnaire is anonymous. You will
find with it a stamped addressed envelope: please
post the questionnaire when completed, if possible
within a week or two of receiving it.

In addition, the Bem Sex Role Inventory (Bem 1974), the
Sex Role Survey (McDonald 1974) and a measure of attitudes toward homosexuality (Weinberg and Williams 1974)
were included. Ten questionnaires from each sample in
which respondents identified themselves were subsequently
compared with interviews with the individuals as a check on
accuracy; no discrepancies were found. Swedish questionnaires were translated into Swedish by two individuals and
checked for accuracy by a third; translation of the Finnish
questionnaire followed a similar procedure. Questionnaires
in Australia and Ireland were in English.

Data Analysis

Analysis was by the χ^2 test for the categorical data and by
Student's t test for the data which had interval or ratio
scales. χ^2 results were calculated on absolute numbers in
all cases, but in some tables row percentages are given to
enable clearer comparisons between countries. Differences
between samples were tested by one-way analysis of variance using post hoc Scheffe tests to determine where any
difference existed.

Results

Sample results are presented in Table 3.1: some differences
were apparent between the samples. Analysis of variance
revealed that there were significant differences between
Australia and Finland on age of the respondents (3.6 years
on average), significant differences in years of education

between Sweden and Ireland (0.8 years on average), and significant differences in number of sexual partners per month over the past year between Sweden and Finland (1.6 per month on average). There were also significant differences between the four countries in terms of the social class of respondents, with more Swedes and Irish reporting that their parents were upper class, and in terms of religious involvement, with more Australians and Irish reporting that they were practicing members of religions.

It is difficult to see how any of the sample differences might affect results. The differences in social class are not paralleled by educational differences, and the age differences are minimal, with only three and a half years difference in mean between the highest and lowest figure. There were no differences between the cultures on age of realization that respondents were homosexual, nor age at which they became homosexually active. There are differences between samples on average number of partners per month. However, the effect of this difference on the data is not clear. The difference on the variable of religion is accounted for in Australia by large congregations of the Metropolitan Community Church, which has a predominantly homosexual congregation. In Ireland, the result is probably due to the influence of the Roman Catholic Church, an organization that is more closely identified with Irish nationality than are churches with nationalism in any of the other three countries from which the samples are derived. Given the substantial similarities between samples, however, and the large number of subjects these data suggest that the four samples are reasonably well matched.

Sample Population, Study Two

The sample consisted of 139 homosexual men in Adelaide, the capital city of South Australia (population 1 million), and was collected in 1984 as part of a prospective study on AIDS. In common with the previous samples, the respondents were comparatively young and well educated, and were recruited by requests for study participants in the local gay magazine, *Catch 22,* notices in two gay bars, the local Metropolitan Community Church, and the local gay sauna, a letter to male members of a gay social club, and requests to the city STD clinic and three city physicians with large homosexual practices to alert patients to the study. The questionnaire was filled out at the same time as respondents had 40 ml of peripheral venous blood taken for determination of mitogenic response and T-cell subsets.

Questionnaire

The questions were part of a wider prospective seroepide-
miological study designed to investigate the factors that
influence the course of AIDs (only one subject was antibody-positive for the HTLV-III virus). Instructions were
as follows:

> As you are probaby aware, there has been a great
> deal of publicity about a number of new and dan-
> gerous diseases in homosexual men overseas, partic-
> ularly AIDS (Acquired Immune Deficiency Syndrome)
> and Kaposi's sarcoma (a form of cancer), and
> Hepatitis B.

> We are undertaking some research to help find out
> which members of the gay population are at risk,
> and what puts them at risk. This will benefit all
> sections of the gay community, not just yourself.
> In order to carry out this research, we need you to
> fill out this questionnaire, and at the same time
> take a blood sample from you. We would also like
> you to provide your name so that if anything
> unusual appears in the blood sample, we can notify
> you. Please provide your name and contact address
> and/or phone number, and sign the form indicating
> that you understand the nature of the study and
> agree to participate.

In addition, five further questionnaires were appended: The
EMBU measure of parental rearing patterns (Perris et al.
1980, Ross, Campbell and Clayer 1982, Ross, Clayer and
Campbell 1983), the short form of the Bem Sex Role Inventory (BSRI) (Andrew and Ross 1982), the Rosenberg Self-
Esteem Scale (Rosenberg 1965) and a measure of homosexual
self-esteem derived from that of Weinberg and Williams
(1974) (Appendix 3). Also included was a measure of
sexual attitudes derived from that developed on heterosexuals by Eysenck (1976) which is illustrated in Appendix
4 and described in detail in Chapter 9, and the Profile of
Mood States (POMS) of McNair, Lorr and Droppleman
(1977).

Data Analysis

Data analysis was by χ^2 test for the categorical data and by
Student's t test for the data that had interval or ratio

scales. One-way analysis of variance using a least-squares difference criterion was used if more than two groups were involved. All χ^2 test were calculated on absolute numbers but in some cases to enable clearer comparisons row percentages are given. Where specific multivariate data analyses peculiar to particular chapters were undertaken, such as linear regressions or factory analyses, these are described in those particular chapters.

Results

Results of the demographic characteristics are presented in Table 3.2. The sample suggests, in common with most research samples of homosexual men, that they are comparatively young and well educated. The number born overseas is not significantly different from the general propulation, but the absence of men of mediterranean origin is of interest. However, in such cultures homosexuals tend not to be open about their sexual orientation, so it is not unexpected that they are not represented in an openly homosexual sample.

As might be expected, the great majority described themselves as exclusively homosexual, although almost one quarter had had heterosexual experience in the past five years. Numbers of sexual partners gave a yearly median figure of 22.6, with the great majority reporting between one and 50. This contrasts markedly with numbers reported in recent United States literature on AIDS, where much higher figures are reported: however, it is debatable whether such figures are representative. The numbers of sexual partners are lower than those reported in the previous Australian sample.

Sexual habits by frequency showed that the most common activity indulged in was oral sex, followed by mutual masturbation; less preferred were anal intercourse (both active and passive) and analingus, which had occurred only in one in five individuals. Sadomasochistic practices were uncommon. Sexual partners were contacted almost equally in bars, discos, or clubs, in the homosexual sauna, cruising, and through friends. The figures for contacts at the sauna may be artificially inflated since some respondents were contacted through this venue. However, these figures refer only to the primary place of contact, and most respondents contacted partners at several locales. Most respondents had been homosexually active for sometime.

Drug use was unremarkable, apart from the almost nonexistent use of hard drugs (opiates or barbiturates).

TABLE 3.2   Demographic Characteristics of the South Australian Sample

Age (Mean ± SD) 33.8 ± 7.8, range 19-54
Education: Tertiary   52.1%
           3 years secondary   28.7%
           3 years secondary   19.2%
Place of birth: Australia   75.0%
                United Kingdom   14.6%
                New Zealand   3.1%
                Other   7.3%
Years in homosexual subculture (mean ± SD) 3.3 ± 2.2, range 0.5-18
Years homosexually active (mean ± SD) 12.8 ± 8.7, range 0.5-38
Sexual partners per month, past year (median) 1.9, range 0-100
Exclusively homosexual: past year   91%
                        past 5 years   76%
Preferred sexual habits: fellatio   71%
                         mutual masturbation   54%
                         anal intercourse--insertor   38%
                         anal intercourse--insertee   35%
                         analingus--active   19%
                         other--brachioproctic   8%
Primary place of contact
for sexual partners: Cruising   27%
                         Friends   21%
                         Sauna   24%
                         Bars, discos, clubs   22%
Drug use, past year: Cigarettes 41.5% (median 20/day)
                         Alcohol (Mean ± SD) - 2.5 ± 2.1 days/week
                                             - 2.5 ± 2.2 glasses/day
                         Marijuana   46.8%
                         Opiates, barbiturates   0.1%
                         Volatile nitrites   30.0%

STD infections:	Past year	Past 5 years
Penile gonorrhea	5	15
Pharyngeal gonorrhea	2	3
Rectal gonorrhea	6	10
Syphillis	1	8
Hepatitis (A, B, non-A, non-B)	2	10
Herpes - lips	11	8
Herpes - penis	4	0
Herpes - anorectal	0	1
Herpes zoster	4	4
Penile warts	2	2
Anorectal warts	1	14
Nongonococcal urethritis	11	23

Hepatitis B surface antibody-positive   36%

The use of alcohol is, however, somewhat above the state average (even considering that South Australia is the main wine growing area of Australia), possibly reflecting the fact that many homosexual social venues serve alcohol.

Incidence of STDs may have been inflated since some respondents were enrolled in the study at the STD clinic or at medical practices. Data showed that 27.3 percent had an STD in the past year if herpes of the lips is excluded, and 63 percent in the past five years also excluding herpes of the lips. Eight respondents had been immunized with hepatitis B vaccine, and 36 percent were hepatitis B surface-antibody positive (similar to the 37 percent reported in the gay sauna by Burrell et al. 1983).

These data suggest that the South Australian sample is comparable to the samples drawn from Queensland and Victoria six years prior to it. However, they also suggest that this sample is different from many reported United States samples, and caution should be used in generalizing to these.

4

Political and Psychosocial Aspects of Homosexual Health Care

In 1982, Altman commented that the "greatest single victory of the gay movement over the past decade has been to shift the debate from behaviour to identity, thus forcing opponents into a position where they can be seen as attacking the civil rights of homosexual citizens rather than attacking specific and (as they see it) antisocial behaviour." Implicit in Altman's observation on the strategy of the gay movement are two other issues of importance: the development of a distinction between homosexual behavior and a homosexual identity, and the development of a connection between homosexuality and politics. Both of these implicit issues need to be elaborated in order to explain how, and why, political beliefs and the health care of homosexual persons are connected. Politics in this sense refers to issues of belief and ideology in an identifiable group of individuals, and in this sense there has really only been a set of politics of homosexuality since there has been an identifiable gay movement.

What are most important in the political aspects of homosexuality are two major developments that parallel, and in fact are implicit in, Altman's comment. First, as the

This chapter is based on the first Michael Q. Petersen Memorial Lecture delivered to the annual conference of the American Physicians for Human Rights, Chicago, August 1984.

focus on the homosexual has shifted from a behavior to an identity, from the individual to the group, it has also shifted from the psychological level in which the focus was on the individual psychopathology, to the political level where the focus is now on the meaning of the identity to the society in which it exists. What was previously a concern of psychiatry and cause for examination of family history for etiologies is now a reason for examining the meaning and control of human sexuality in society.

Second, the development of a public homosexual identity has meant that within the homosexual community there has developed a diversity (recognized by Bell and Weinberg in the title of their 1978 publication, Homosexualities) of lifestyle as well as attitudes toward sexual orientation and its meaning. As a consequence, it is possible to identify a number of different beliefs about homosexuality, its relationship with society, and its meaning to the individual. These attitudes and meanings are probably central to the political aspects of health care in homosexuals both because they tend to covary with important variables including expression of sexuality (such as partner numbers) and psychological factors (such as self-image).

This final point also raises a third question that needs to be answered if the health care of homosexuals can become a subject of meaningful debate. How is the health care of homosexuals different from that of heterosexuals? The answer is that there are two major areas in which homosexual men may differ from nonhomosexuals. First, as Ross, Rogers and McCulloch (1978) have observed, the only thing in the final analysis that distinguishes homosexuals from heterosexuals is the degree and form of social stigmatization to which they may be subject. This has its clearest implications for mental health, particularly matters of self-esteem and depression and anxiety, but also has implications for psychosomatic disorders such as gastrointestinal ulceration and hypertension.

Second, as has been apparent from the emphasis in several recent books on health care and homosexuals, homosexuals differ from nonhomosexuals in their incidence of sexually related disease. In the case of males, homosexual men have a generally higher incidence than heterosexual men: in the case of lesbians, the incidence is lower than in heterosexual women. Of interest in this context is also the fact that Freedman (1971) found that lesbians had *less* psychological adjustment difficulties than heterosexual women; it may be that being a lesbian is a protection against psychological difficulties and sexually related diseases. For this reason, and because most of the available data are on males, the situation of the male homosexual is discussed here.

However, it is necessary to be more specific about why and how sexually transmitted diseases are more prevalent in some sectors of the homosexual community: there are probably three specific causes. Increases in partner numbers are likely to lead to increased risks of contracting infection. Increases in partners met at places for anonymous encounters such as baths and back-room bars are likely to bring together individuals with high partner numbers, producing a multiplicative effect for risk of transmission of infection, as well as decreasing the possibility of contact tracing. Parenthetically, the importance of contact tracing in bringing to treatment asymptomatic carriers is probably underestimated, as well as the chance to treat subsequent contacts before they have infected too many other individuals. The third cause is the actual sexual practices which are favored: for example, the risks of brachioproctic practices ("fist-fucking") and probably insertee anal intercourse are greater than, for example, mutual masturbation or frottage.

Do political beliefs affect homosexual and lesbian health care? If political beliefs are defined not in terms of party political identification, or liberalism and conservatism, but as views on the meaning of homosexuality in a society, the answer must be yes. There are in fact three avenues in which health care may be affected: through external pressures such as the attitudes of community and government to gay clinics, in the community's attitude toward homosexuality, and in the subsequent funding and support of health care for sexual minorities. This form of influence is perhaps the most obvious and well documented, and need not be elaborated on here. The second involves the political attitudes of the homosexual patient or potential patient, in the sense that these attitudes will be related to such risk factors as partner numbers, partner anonymity, sexual practices, and self-image. The third variable is the physician, whose attitudes to homosexual patients will vary not only if the physician is a heterosexual, but also if she or he is homosexual and their own attitudes toward homosexuality in society. These last two groups, the patient and the physician, will be examined in turn.

When we talk of political factors in the health care of homosexual men and lesbians, then, we are ultimately talking about how political beliefs come to be reflected in health-related behaviors. The mechanism is probably one of both political beliefs and the social or societal imposition of frameworks in which homosexuality is seen, along with initially unrelated factors such as beliefs about health and illness influencing behavior. Societal factors are also going to be important in their own right in that individuals in societies or situations that are antihomosexual, and greater stresses if they have to hide their sexual orientation—very much a Catch 22 situation. Under such conditions, then it is most likely that higher stress will lead to higher auto- nomic arousal and that there will be a higher incidence of stress and arousal-related disorders such as gastrointestinal disturbances, respiratory problems, migraine, hypertension, and the effects of stress on the immune system. One of the barriers to gay health care is probably the fact that the connection is not made often enough between a gay lifestyle and inherently nonsexual aspects of health. Too often physicians, and more frequently patients, do not attempt to modify lifestyle in order to control physical problems—and this includes such problems as smoking and alcohol and drug abuse, which may have significant lifestyle components. In some cases, simple counseling by the physician can help the patient to make connections between stress, behavior, and illness and modify some of the con- tributors. Given that the source of the stress is clearly external and does not involve placing any blame on, or inducing any guilt in, the patient, this may act as a trig- ger for better understanding of gay health problems that are not seen as being explicitly related to homosexuality.

However, perhaps the most important political aspect of gay health care is the relationship between political beliefs ("world views") and health-related behaviors. Homosexu- ality is something that can be seen as having different political and social statuses and roles in Western society: for example, while some writers believe that it is an orien- tation that calls into question the basic organizational unit of modern society, the family, and the sexist stratification of modern culture (and thus is a force for radical social change), others hold conflicting views. The so-called revisionists believe, on the contrary, that while homosex- uality does raise a number of questions about individuals' rights and moral values in modern society, the society in which we exist is soundly based and requires change from within and in its detail rather than in totality. Yet a third tradition holds that the overall organization of society has been imposed and that the individual will hold within herself or himself the knowledge and ability to make moral decisions about the organization of his or her own lifestyle and relationships.

Each of these three traditions has important implications for how homosexuality fits or does not fit into Western society and thus the meaning of homosexual behavior. It is these different meanings that will affect the individual's attitudes toward relationships, sex roles, sexual behaviors, partner numbers, and sexually related diseases. It will in all probability affect the way such individuals see their own homosexuality and thus their mental health. Can such dimensions of political belief be demonstrated in homosexuals? Do they have consequences for health and health care? If this can be empirically demonstrated, we are well on the way to including political factors as important covariates with homosexual and homosocial behavior and identity and consequences with gay health risks and health care.

Attitudes to political institutions and to society have not previously been measured, and it is not difficult to see why. Measuring beliefs about what society is for, and how it works and should be organized, are to a degree equivalent to asking individuals what the meaning of life is, since their perception of how they fit into society and their goals may well depend on this. To a homosexual individual, asking what being homosexual or being attracted to members of the same sex means is broaching much the same issues, and it has considerable implications for health care in homosexual men and women. The reason for this is that sexuality, and particularly sexual behavior, occurs within a social as well as an interpersonal context, and both the behavior and the individual's self-image will depend on where they see sexuality fitting into society. For example, if an individual sees a homosexual orientation as being a statement against society and a symbol of an alternative type of interaction or social structure, then that individual's sexual behavior will probably be driven by a desire to express this to society, as well as by personal needs. On the other hand, if an individual sees a homosexual orientation as being simply another variation within a range tolerated to a greater or lesser extent by society, and antihomosexual attitudes as being peculiar to particular religious and moral viewpoints, then that individual will probably tend to deemphasize their sexuality or keep it in line with prevailing norms. There is probably a third alternative, which is seeing sexuality as being a variable unrelated to the structure or function of society and a matter of individual choice or preference, and in this situation the individual's sexuality will probably be a matter of personal needs and views to a much larger extent than in the previous two examples. Nevertheless, such personal needs and views themselves will also be colored by the society in which the individual lives and society's reaction to homosexual behavior. The fourth alternative is of course acceptance of the belief that homosexual behavior threatens the status quo and the fabric of society, and this would probably lead to a lower and more guilt-ridden level of sexual behavior, as well as relatively severe psychological consequences such as lack of self-acceptance and increased tension.

Can dimensions such as these be demonstrated to occur in homosexual men? Israel (1972) has noted that in all theory, assumptions about the nature of humans and society are implicit; in fact, he argues that they are stipulative assumptions at a prescientific level and form the basis of social organization. If it is assumed that there is an interaction between political beliefs about society and attitudes (Figure 4.1), in that people tend to see things in the way that they categorize them, behavior is thus created in accordance with what is assumed in a form of self-fulfilling prophecy. Taking Israel's suggestion a step further, it becomes apparent that the various statements of sociological theorists are normative and not descriptive statements. If this is the case, then differing views of society, and its goals, functions, and norms should also correspond with attitudes and behaviors, including sexual ones.

Figure 4.1

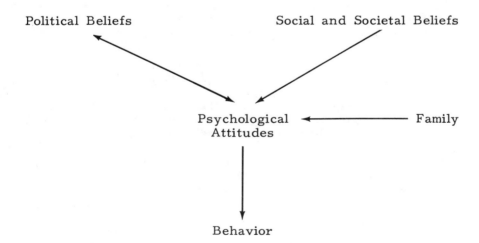

Three models of society can be described in terms of both function and structure. Functional models include mechanistic views, in which society is seen as a closed

system seeking equilibrium; organic models see social systems as a set of clearly differentiated elements stressing an
objective normality and set structures; and process models
view society as a complex and multifaceted interplay under-
going continuous development. The more widely recognized
structural models (which Israel argues are in fact normative
prescriptions) are the consensus and conflict models. The
consensus model is described by Wild (1978) as seeing
"society as an organism that tries to maintain itself in some
kind of equilibrium by the harmonious functioning of its
various parts. Stability and order are seen as natural and
normal, whereas conflict and disorder are viewed as deviant
phenomena which show that the system is not working
correctly." Equality is seen to be unachievable, and the
system is regarded as the best possible. Altman (1971)
sees this, in the homosexual context, as similar to the
attitude of some older homosexuals who have already established a way of coping with the world—to such people, he
suggests, the concept of gay liberation is as much a threat
as it is to heterosexual society because it undermines the
whole complex set of roles, social relationships, and assimilation strategies set up by such individuals.

In contrast, the conflict model "views society as a loose
collection of institutions, controlled and dominated by those
in power. . . . The powerful . . . control others through
institutionalised and ideological dominance. . . . Conflict is
seen as inherent and natural in social organisation and
greater equality is achievable" (Wild 1978). In terms of the
impact of homosexuality on Western society, Altman (1971)
notes that seen in this light, homosexuality has come to
represent a challenge to conventional norms that thus make
the homosexual a revolutionary. The implication of homosexuality is to provide a catalyst to break out and become
free, and to work for fundamental changes in the institutions that oppress people such as the family system, and
sex typing. For change in any basic system, changes must
be made in related ones such as education, economics, and
law. Thus, at least two contrasting models of society have
been traditionally posited: Altman considers that the differences between them, at the level of homosexual organizations, is equivalent to the difference between liberal pressure groups as against a revolutionary attitude. If these
models are to be of any use in empirically demonstrating
that political and social views do influence homosexual
health- and sexuality-related behaviors, then we must not
only demonstrate that such dimensions exist but that they
are significantly related to sexual expression. The study
which follows is based on these two hypotheses.

METHOD

In an attempt to elucidate what dimensions of societal process and structure could be differentiated, 50 items, that dealt with various domains of social model including mechanistic, organic, process, static versus dynamic, ultimate control by majority, anarchistic, and conflict versus stability were generated. These were given to 176 Swedish homosexual men in 1977 in Stockholm, as part of a wider study of male homosexuality in Sweden: sample characteristics are provided in Table 3.1 in Chapter 3.

Factor analysis (oblique rotation) of these items lead to eight interpretable factors being extracted. These factors included, as the first three, which accounted for over 50 percent of the common variance between them, described dimensions of consensus and need for order (Factor 1), belief in conflict and constant change (Factor 2), and a belief in individual's rights to determine their own lifestyles (Factor 3). These factors (Table 4.1) are referred to as the Consensus-Order, Conflict, and Anarchy factors. When they are factor-scored, they may be compared as dimensions with other variables including the attitudes of the respondents to relationships and roles within relationships, attitude toward their own homosexuality, actual and expected societal reaction to their homosexuality from significant others, demographic variables such as age, education, class, and position on the Kinsey Scale, and personality variables such as masculinity (instrumental behavior and dominance) and femininity (expressive behavior and passivity) on the Bem Sex Role Inventory.

RESULTS AND DISCUSSION

Results of correlations between the three political dimensions and attitudinal, demographic, and personality variables are presented in Tables 4.2–4.4 and confirm that not only are there empirically demonstrable dimensions of societal perception in the Swedish homosexual men who filled out the questionnaire, but also that they are significantly related to attitudes and behaviors that have health-care implications. These health-care implications are particularly in the areas of sexually transmitted diseases (STDs) and mental health.

Reference to Table 4.2 illustrates that a large and internally coherent set of variables correlates significantly with the Consensus for Order factor. First, the strength of the dimension increases with age, paralleling a known

TABLE 4.1 First Three Factors Derived from Beliefs about Society Questionnaire

---

FACTOR 1: Consensus for Order   Factor Loading

21   In any society, some people will be more equal than others.   .59
26   When most people in a society agree, one has
       achieved the goal.   .52
17   Order is vitally important for any society of harmony.   .47
23   Society should have clear norms or patterns for people
       to follow.   .47
 9   People who disagree with society should try to adapt
       to a majority decision.   .40
37   Governments should ultimately be responsible for controlling
       people's actions.   .37
 5   Even when we disagree with the majority, we should go
       along with their choice.   .36
                        (30% of variance)

FACTOR 2: Conflict

10   A certain degree of conflict in a society is desirable.   .51
11   Sometimes, individual rights should be limited for the
       good of society.   -.51
 7   Conflict is normal in a well-adjusted society.   .44
30   Constant change in any society is a good thing.   .42
12   If people don't want to do things for their society,
       they shouldn't be forced to.   .40
                        (12% of variance)

FACTOR 3: Anarchist

12   If people don't want to do things for their society,
       they shouldn't be forced to.   .67
 4   A person should have the right to live in disorder if
       they want to.   .51
34   We need strong laws to keep order in society.   -.37
16   Societies should be as open to change from outside factors
       as from inside ones.   .36
                        (10% of variance)

---

relationship between increasing age and increasing conservatism. It also increases with religious attachment as
would be expected given the strong support conventional
Christian denominations provide for the established social

TABLE 4.2 Consensus--Order Correlations

- Increases with age (.23)
- Increases with religious attachment (.34)
- Increases with defining self as more heterosexual (.14)
- More likely to play male-female roles (.34)
- More likely to play dominant-submissive roles (.32)
- These roles more likely to be rigid (.23)
- Believe gay relationships should be only between two people, not more (.23)
- More likely to have had negative reaction to homosexuality (.21) and less likely to expect negative reaction (1.14)
- Less likely to have high partner numbers (-.14)

---

order both through moral pronouncements and support for current social structures. In terms of the degree of homosexuality as measured on the Kinsey Scale, high Consensus and Order scorers tend to describe themselves as more heterosexual, an interesting finding as it suggests that they are either attempting to define themselves as more in the predominant sexual orientation (so-called "defense bisexuals"), or that they are actually more bisexual and thus identify more with the predominant and socially sanctioned form of sexual expression.

In terms of data on beliefs and practices about roles and role playing in homosexual relationships, those scoring high on the Consensus-Order dimension are significantly more likely to play "male-female" and dominant-submissive roles in a gay relationship, and these roles are more likely to be rigid ones that do not vary across situations. Again, these data confirm that those who believe that society has a right to extract conformity tend to mimic dominant societal values and accept them as universal truths (in this case, the dominance of the heterosexual and male-female status differential model). In an echo of this, we see that high scorers on the Consensus-Order dimension believe that relationships should be exclusively between two people: strongly supporting this, the data also show that Consensus-Order supporters are less likely to have high partner numbers.

Perception of society and its reaction to homosexuality is perhaps central to demonstrating the concurrent validity of the Consensus-Order dimension. On the measure of actual reaction from significant others to the respondent's homosexual orientation, high Consensus-Order individuals are *more likely to have had* a negative reaction, but *less likely to expect* such a reaction. Thus such individuals tend to see society and significant others as more accepting of homosexuality despite personal experience to the contrary. Generally, then, the high Consensus-Order respondents have what could be described as more conservative attitudes to sexual relationships and see them in a fairly heterosexual model. Of particular importance for health-related behaviors is the fact that sexual expression is not seen as a factor setting homosexual individuals apart from society, and thus not strongly emphasized: high Consensus-Order scorers tend to see themselves within a general relational model in which gender of partner is not of central importance to the structure and conduct of the relationship. Thus, partner numbers appear to be comparatively low, and belief in less negative societal reaction to homosexuality will be associated with better mental health (Ross 1978).

The second dimension extracted is entitled the Conflict dimension, and again presents a coherent set of items (Table 4.3) that indicate that high scorers on this dimension believe that conflict is desirable and normal in society, that constant change in society is good, and that individuals should not be forced to do things in support of a society they may not agree with. Similarly, high Conflict dimension scorers disagree that there are any grounds for limiting individual rights, since this would presumably limit the potential for change and suppress conflict. As with the Consensus-Order dimension, the Conflict dimension contains a coherent set of items with homosexual behavior and attitude interrelationships.

TABLE 4.3 Conflict Correlations

- No gay relationship 2 years (.13)
- Believe gay relationships should be sexual only (.21)
- Believe relationships for gays not natural (.15)
- More likely to be less accepting of own homosexuality (.26)
- Likely to be lower on dominance-assertiveness (.14)
- Likely to have high partner numbers (.14)

The perceptions of relationships in the high Conflict scorers are very different to those of the Consensus-Order high scorers. High-Conflict-scoring individuals are less likely to have had a homosexual relationship which lasted more than two years, believe gay relationships should be sexual only, and believe that for homosexuals, relationships are not natural (presumably because they are a heterosexual model and thus are a result of identification with the aggressor). Of particular interest is the fact that high Conflict scorers are likely to be less accepting of their own homosexuality, perhaps due to their seeing it as being very much at odds with the dominant ethic of the society in which they live: the role of the revolutionary is said to be always hard and demanding, and self-doubt may not be uncommon.

Other associations with high Conflict scores are lower scores on the masculinity measuring (dominance-assertiveness) scale—possibly an artifact of the fact that rejection of the masculine norm leads to individuals rating themselves as more feminine (expressive) and, of central importance, high Conflict scorers are likely to have higher partner numbers. This last point is of importance in its implications for health care. It suggests that individuals with the political view that homosexuality acts as a lifestyle that confronts and challenges society and societal bases, such as patriarchal organization and the nuclear family, have higher partner numbers. As such, expression of one's sexuality becomes a visible way of confronting society (particularly since homosexual persons are defined primarily in terms of sexual acts) and of expressing opposition to the current system. What is being described is essentially homosexual sex as a revolutionary act, and those who most strongly believe that society is a conflict-based system in which change is essential will be those most likely to view homosexual sex as a highly cathected act. Since such individuals also tend to reject the idea that homosexual relationships (other than sexual ones) are appropriate, they are at higher health risk for sexually related diseases due to both higher partner numbers as well as probably a greater degree of anonymous sex. Similarly, such individuals are probably also at greater risk in mental health terms as a result of feeling less accepting of their own homosexuality as well as tending to see themselves as a minority battling against the mores and values of a rejecting and often punitive society that they are in but not part of.

The third dimension extracted from the Swedish sample is the Anarchy factor. In contrast to the previous dimensions of Consensus-Order and Conflict, the Anarchy dimension measures individual's beliefs in basic human rights to differ and to be at variance with the dominant societal model if they so wish. In many ways the Anarchy dimension is opposed to the Consensus-Order dimension since the Consensus-Order dimensions sees order and stability as being important while the Anarchy dimension sees it as irrelevant to the individual. Altman (1971) has in fact commented of the homosexual situation that "Only Socialism highly flavoured by Anarchism would seem consistent with sexual liberation." Thus, high Anarchy scorers (Table 4.4) believe that individuals shouldn't be forced to work within society if they don't want to, should have the right to live outside the conventional norms without being forced into line by laws or social pressure, and that societies should be open to change from all directions. Perhaps the best description of high Anarchy scorers is that they are not bound by rigid social models of any sort, but tend to be internally controlled by their own beliefs and values. If society and their values should conflict, then their values would be taken as the most important: the impression gained is that high Anarchy scorers would support the situational ethic rather than any set of rules that was prescriptive. This picture is supported by the items correlating with high Anarchy scores: as beliefs in Anarchy increase, so does educational attainment, and concommitantly religious attachment decreases.

TABLE 4.4 Anarchy Correlations

- Increases with education (.17)
- Decreases with religious attachment (.18)
- Believe gay relationships should be sexual only (.17)
- Less likely to differentiate domestic roles in relationship (.15)
- More likely to believe that relationships for gays not natural (.14)

In common with the Conflict model, the Anarchy model supporters believe that gay relationships should be sexual only and that they are not natural: on the other hand, there is *no* relationship with partner numbers or with self-acceptance as homosexual, which suggests that the sexual activity the individual prefers is related to situations and times rather than seen as a political statement with implications for social change. The high Anarchy scorers are also less likely to differentiate homosexual relationships when they are in them, which suggests that they are not role bound but able to accept people as individuals rather than as symbols of societal structures.

These three groups of political attitudes clearly have

implications for sexual behavior and as a consequence for health in homosexual men and women. Whether personality affects political attitudes, in the sense that people choose political stances that best fit their attitudes and activities, or whether the reverse is true and political attitudes affect behavior and attitudes, cannot be determined: probably, like most situations, there is an interactive effect. Nevertheless, the link between political beliefs and attitudes toward homosexual identities and behaviors is, if not accounting for a great proportion of variance, consistent and clearly demonstrable. What it does emphasize most strongly is how within a homosexual population there are a number of dimensions of political beliefs—beliefs in what homosexual identities and behaviors mean to them—that may have very considerable health-care implications. Such implications include direct variables such as partner numbers and probably anonymity of partners, as well as indirect variables such as the meanings of sexual encounters, sexually related diseases, treatment, and the mental health consequences of particular beliefs about a homosexual orientation.

In terms of treatment, there is a real dilemma about how health professionals should react to the relationship of political beliefs and health-related behaviors. It is clear that in contrast to most other minority groups, homosexual women and men bring a very different set of political perceptions to their stigmatization. While ethnic and racial minorities have both a cultural history and identity that is able to be transmitted through the family, and share a common unit of social organization in the family, a homosexual orientation provides neither a basic social unit that is identical to that in the dominant culture nor an alternative culture or belief system that is handed down via such a social unit. The social pressures on homosexual men and women are thus different in kind from those faced by cultural minorities and there is little history and few roles to guide them other than those largely negative and inaccurate ones passed down by the heterosexual majority. The position of women may be a better model, although they are not of course a minority and do have a form of culture, however inappropriate, expressed in roles and passed on through families. Nevertheless, the political perceptions of minority status in homosexual women and men will be different in that it has to be supplied rather than is provided, and in that it has very few points of assimilation into the dominant culture apart from converting itself into a mimicry of heterosexual marriage. Under such conditions of strong dissimilarity, the political implications of a homosexual identity are emphasized.

IMPLICATIONS FOR HEALTH CARE

Where these political beliefs have health implications, should health professionals attempt to modify them? The enormous dangers of altering an individual's most precious and most important beliefs precludes any modification of the way the individual sees the world, since it would be equivalent to attempting to remove a personality or religious belief, or any other central guiding principle. It would also be equivalent to removing the individual's carefully built-up understanding of gay culture, although to many gay individuals this may seem to be unconsciously absorbed and independent of any "political" view. However, as has already been demonstrated, there is an implied political viewpoint in any perception of the homosexual person, particularly in homosexual persons themselves.

What is preferable to any modification of attitudes or meanings of homosexual identities or behaviors is making individuals aware of the health consequences of their attitudes. Frequently the health professional will accept without implied or actual criticism from a homosexual person descriptions of health risks that should be discussed: this may occur particularly if the physician is himself or herself homosexual. There is no implied criticism in leading the patient to an *awareness* of the relationship between political or social attitudes and health risks. On the other hand, if the individual is well aware of the risks of some particular behavior, then it may be inappropriate to stress the importance of health and safety as if they are the only aspects of lifestyle that are important. Nevertheless, it is not uncommon for individuals to deny health risks because the cessation of particular behaviors (whether they be cruising in dangerous areas, potentially dangerous practices such as "fist-fucking," or multiple partners in short time spans, or rejecting treatment advice) is too threatening or the behaviors concerned are too strongly cathected, driven or otherwise central to self-image. In such cases, the practitioner may well have the option of discussing the meaning of such behaviors and providing the patient with an awareness of, and insight into, the linkage between attitude, belief, and behavior. Insight provided in such a way may be the only stimulus needed to induce lower risks. On the other hand, perception of degree of risk (a concept whereby in many cases in homosexual health care there is little consistent evidence and much inconsistent opinion) may be based more on the health professional's political attitudes and beliefs, and the critical interface of social and political values that occurs between patient and physician.

THE PHYSICIAN AND SOCIOPOLITICAL
ASPECTS OF HEALTH CARE OF HOMOSEXUALS

Without doubt, the reaction of the attending health-care professional to the homosexual patient is, as the other side of the equation of gay and lesbian health care, of equal importance in discussing the barriers and inducements to treatment and compliance. In fact, the politicization of the gay medical profession has been one of the major positive aspects of the homosexual liberation movements, and appears to fit surprisingly well with the model of development of sexual identity described by Cass (1979). Cass' model posits six stages of the development of a homosexual identity in the individual: Identity Confusion, Identity Comparison, Identity Tolerance, Identity Acceptance, Identity Pride, and Identity Synthesis. Identity Confusion describes the stage where individuals feel they are different from others and that their feelings or behaviors may be labeled as homosexual. For the medical profession, this stage is equivalent to a vague awareness that health-care needs for homosexual and heterosexual people may be different, but not acting on this. The second stage, Identity Comparison, is for the individual the first tentative commitment to a homosexual identity: for the homosexual physician, it represents an awareness that distinctions may be made between conventional practices and those that seem to attract more homosexual or bisexual individuals. In this situation, the ability to differentiate between typically heterosexual and specifically homosexual difficulties becomes more marked as the physician sees more homosexual patients.

With Identity Tolerance in the individual, the third stage of the Cass model, comes the recognition that she or he is probably homosexual, and a degree of commitment to this identity arises. For the gay physician, this stage is probably marked by the increasing recognition that their practice is predominantly gay, and a degree of commitment to gay patients. Contact with other gay physicians may occur. By stage four, the Identity Acceptance stage, the individual accepts the label of homosexual, at least in gay company, and begins to socialize within a gay subculture. For the physician, this stage probably represents the acceptance of the fact that the practice is homosexually oriented and admission or advertisement of this within certain limited social confines. The stage of Identity Pride for an individual is marked by wide disclosure and open activism, and for homosexual physicians this represents openly advertising as a homosexual physician and joining in public association with others (such as Bay Area Physicians, American Association of Physicians for Human Rights, and Australian Gay Medical Association). This is probably the present stage for the organization of the gay medical practitioner: the recognition of homosexual health care as a speciality and pride in this fact.

The sixth stage of the Cass model is perhaps the one that has stimulated most debate. In the individual, the "them versus us" view of homosexuals and heterosexuals fades, and is replaced by a situation where the person's homosexual identity is seen as being one of a series of identities, but not one that defines all aspects of the lifestyle. What might this correspond to in the case of homosexual health-care providers? I suspect that its closest equivalent is the recognition that sexually related diseases are only part of the health care of homosexual individuals, and that in many cases there are fewer differences between homosexual and heterosexual health care than were initially imagined. At this point, perhaps, emphasis may shift toward psychosomatic illnesses, and other risk factors of a gay lifestyle where these exist (such as smoking, alcohol, and drugs, as well as matters of diet and fitness). Perhaps even the sexual orientation may even be seen as unimportant for many points of consultation or referral. This, however, is to a degree speculative, but there is no doubt that Cass' model of sexual identification does provide a useful framework to examine the progressive development of homosexual health care on the part of medical practitioners in a political and social context, and thus to map the barriers and advantages in terms of the physician's contribution to homosexual health care.

A further sociopolitical consideration affecting health care in the homosexual community is the *distribution* of practices or clinics specializing in homosexual health care. These tend to be concentrated in larger cities where there are identifiable homosexual communities, and in larger cities where there are identifiable homosexual communities, and in larger cities they tend to be clustered around the so-called "gay ghettos" in which a number of homosexual men (and frequently women) are domiciled within a small area. Thus, the gay clinics have tended to develop in areas in which homosexual people who follow the homosexual identity/homosexual culture definition of their orientation will make up a large proportion of the practice (for example, Castro Street and Polk Street in San Francisco). The effect of this is twofold: first, the practice population tends to be those for whom homosexuality is a central aspect of their definition (in Cass' model, those at the stage of homosexual pride) and thus for whom self-esteem is being built and probably a high number of sexual partners are being enjoyed. Second, this emphasis on a homosexual identity suggests that the patients to such a practice will tend to see homosexual health care only in genital or sexual terms, and other aspects of health care as unrelated to lifestyle. While this is probably an overgeneralization, it illustrates the point that homosexual health care should not be assumed to apply only to those whose sexuality is a central definition of their lifestyle, and whose concerns and problems are going to be different from those who Cass describes in her model as stage 4 (Identity Acceptance), and those at stage 6 (Identity Synthesis), in which homosexual behavior has probably superceded homosexual identity. In accepting social, political, and psychological dimensions to homosexual behaviors and identities, and that individuals may ascribe different meanings and emphases to their sexuality at different points of their development, it must not be assumed that geographical concentrations that tend to cluster particular world views of sexual orientation and stages of identity are all that homosexual health care is about. It is equally important that the smaller North American, European, and Australian cities without highly developed gay foci are seen as presenting different but equally important forms of health care, although they may have different distributions of homosexual identity development, different legal responses to same-sex behavior, and different presenting problems in quality, quantity, and type. Physicians staffing such practices will also tend to fall within the analogous stages of Cass' model as applied to gay medical identity, most probably further down the scale as centers of population get smaller and attitudes to homosexuality more rigid.

This conceptualization of the points of identity of the patient and the health professional, and the degree of correspondence or mismatch between them, defines a further barrier to gay and lesbian health care in which practitioner and patient are equal contributors. If a table were to be drawn up looking at physicians whose political beliefs about homosexuality were plotted against patient's political beliefs about homosexuality (Table 4.5), it would be apparent that any one of the nine possible combinations of physician and patient beliefs about the political meaning of homosexuality could have a different effect. If one looks at the leading diagonal in which the patient's and physician's views are congruent, then what is going to occur is reinforcement of both of the participant's views of homosexuality, with positive implications for transference and counter-trans-

TABLE 4.5 Possible Interactions Between Political Views of Physician and Patient

Patient Views	Physician Views		
	Consensus	Conflict	Anarchy
Consensus-Order	Reinforce	Disagree	Agree
Conflict	Disagree	Reinforce	Agree
Anarchy	Agree/ Disagree	Agree/ Disagree	Reinforce

ference. In situations where there is a clear dichotomy between the views of physician and patient, for example where the physician is a high Consensus-Order dimension scorer and the patient a high Conflict dimension scorer or the converse, there is the potential for disagreement and negative transference and counter-transference. Given that one of the bases of successful counseling and consultation is accurate empathy with the client (Truax and Carkhuff 1967), and that accurate empathy is severely hampered by fundamentally opposing conceptions of one of the central issues for consultation, then it must be recognized that a potential barrier to health care includes disjunction of concepts of the problem. In the case of a physician who is a high scorer on the Anarchy dimension, then the view that it is the patient's right to see her or his sexual orientation in any way they please is going to provide acceptance of almost any social or political perception of a homosexual identity. In fact, it is probable that a majority of physicians with predominantly homosexual practices fall into this category. For the reverse situation in which the patient is a high Anarchy dimension scorer but the physician is a believer in either the Consensus-Order or Conflict views of homosexual identity, then the result will be either agreement or disagreement depending on the presenting problem and what it reveals to the attending physician about the patient's background and views.

While this model of physician-patient interaction has been presented in an extreme form to clarify it, the principles of the interaction are the important aspect, particularly with regard to transference and counter-transference problems that are the actual barriers to appropriate health care. Nor need the model used be one of political dimensions: the six stages of the Cass model of homosexual identity formation could equally easily be substituted into the grid, or attitudes to homosexuality by nonhomosexual practitioners dealing with gay patients, or any variation on these themes. The critical point is that it is as much a barrier to health care to have disagreement within the homosexual patient-physician diad as it is to have it within the diad of the nonhomosexual physician and patient, and unless we become aware of this it will become a significant barrier to health care. It is probably as naive to imagine that the conception and conduct of homosexual behavior or homosexual identity is homogeneous within homosexual groups or individuals any more than it is for heterosexuals. As a consequence, within homosexual communities (although on a much restricted scale compared to attitudes to and conceptions of homosexual activity within the heterosexual community) variations will occur that have implications for health care if they occur between physician and patient.

The mechanism for such health care barriers occurs through the mechanisms of transference and counter-transference. In the situation where an orientation such as a homosexual one is stigmatized, the potential for positive transference between a homosexual patient and their physician is greatly enhanced: likewise, the counter-transference from physician to patient is also likely to be enhanced as a function of the identification of each other as accepting, understanding, and similar in sexuality and probably a great deal more. The effect of this positive transference or counter-transference may pose some dangers, particularly if the physician believes that homosexual individuals have suffered sufficiently at the hands of a rejecting society and does not question aspects of the patient's health-related behaviors that might be raised. Perhaps an analogy is the case of the health professional who is a heavy smoker and who does not raise questions about the dangers of smoking in a patient. A second issue is whether seeing homosexual health as relating solely to sexual matters in only reinforcing the perception of homosexuality as an essentialized condition, and avoiding non-sexual health consequences of lifestyle. With positive counter-transference the physician may well wish not to raise matters that might be construed to be a criticism of a homosexual identity rather than a questioning of some of the consequences of lifestyle for health and illness. Conversely in the case of negative counter-transference, the physician's criticisms may be construed by the patient in much more negative terms and have the effect of lowering their self-esteem or their self-acceptance of their homosexual orientation. Should this occur at an early stage of homosexual identity development, for example in a situation where an individual is at the stage of coming out and experimenting with a new lifestyle, particularly in terms of high partner numbers, it may severely compromise the development of a homosexual identity. Perhaps the best solution may involve careful exploration of the reasons for particular behaviors that may be potentially hazardous, and the motivations behind and the meanings attached to them. Only after such careful probing is it possible to determine whether discussions about risks involved will have a negative or a positive effect on the patient, and whether the behaviors might be modifiable or warnings given. In the event that behaviors appear not to be modifiable or there are not viable alternatives, then education of the patient is often the most appropriate option, and it is probable that no physician uses as much of this alternative as he or she might. Where a high-risk behavior occurs, and will continue to occur, it is possible to inform patients of ways to minimize risk and to become aware of dangerous consequences as early as possible and to seek treatment as soon as possible.

As an example of this latter approach, if a patient is so involved in brachioproctic eroticism ("fist-fucking") that he or she is not prepared to forego this activity, education about risk factors and how to modify them is essential (for example, lubricants, cutting finger-nails, avoiding the extension of digits, avoiding partners who are under the influence of drink or drugs and avoiding taking part in such activities while under the influence of agents that might mask signs of injury, learning the early symptoms of bowel perforation and peritonitis, and the urgency of early treatment).

Ultimately, health care in the homosexual person as in any other group involves an interaction between physician and patient, and while patient factors probably account for a greater proportion of the variation in health risk than do physician factors, we cannot afford to ignore our own roles as health professionals in modification and education as well as treatment or the interactive effects of our social and political stances with those of our patients. Not only may the consequences be worse for the already stigmatized gay individual, but the awareness of potential areas of difficulty may also help to avoid unnecessary barriers to homosexual health care. The enormous variation within those with a homosexual orientation makes it important to recognize that while in many ways this provides any homosexual community with advantages, from the point of view of assuming that homosexuality equals homogeneity it adds another dimension of risk and further potential barriers and opportunities to homosexual health care.

5

Correlates of Number of Sexually Transmitted Disease Infections: A Psychoepidemiological Study

There has been very little research to date on the social and epidemiological correlates of STD infections in heterosexual individuals, and virtually none on homosexual men. Indeed, it is fairly clear from the previous research reviewed in Chapter 2 that it is dangerous to make generalizations from heterosexual STD correlates to homosexual ones for several reasons. This is because, first, homosexuality is still socially stigmatized and this stigmatization may directly or indirectly promote behaviors that increase the risk of STD infection. Second, sexual activities in homosexual men are generally likely to be different in type to those most commonly performed in a heterosexual context (although with the exception of penovaginal intercourse, all sexual acts that are performed by homosexual men may be performed by heterosexual couples). Third, homosexual samples are most commonly biased by being composed disproportionately of better educated and thus less working class individuals, in contrast to the studies of STDs in heterosexuals that tend to have the opposite bias: as a consequence educational and class variation is liable to be misinterpreted as variation due to sexual orientation. Fourth, it is probable that attitudes toward sexuality and views of the function of sexuality are different between (or for that matter, within) homosexuals and heterosexuals and that this may radically alter determinants of sexual behavior.

Thus, the absence of any strong guidelines from previous research on heterosexuals and lack of information on homosexual men makes it imperative to carry out a basic epidemiological study on the factors that appear to contribute to STD infection. Since prospective studies are expensive and time consuming, the most appropriate form of epidemiological study is the case-control method, in which we compare those who have contracted STDs with those who have not, and then examine those variables which discriminate these groups. Where there are discriminators, they should provide clues as to what variables appear to be associated with STD infection and how the association affects (or is affected by) infection. The second stage of such research involves looking at the specific variables implicated in some detail to establish how and why they may affect whether the individual does or does not become infected. A third stage, the most difficult, time consuming, and expensive, is the intervention study in which one manipulates the putative precursors of STD infections and follows through the subjects over a period of time to determine if the manipulation was effective or not.

This book does not include intervention studies but will hopefully provide background data that provide the empirical bases for experimental verification. Until the occurrence of acquired immune deficiency syndrome (AIDS), in fact, STDs in homosexual men (or any other individuals) would not have been regarded as a sufficiently severe condition to attempt intervention: as already noted in Chapter 2, STDs were seen by some individuals as a desirable punishment to enforce prevailing moral standards or double standards.

The aim of this chapter is to provide answers to two questions. First, what are the social and psychological variables associated with STD infections in homosexual men that are common across Western societies? Second, what do the social and psychological variables that are specific to particular countries tell us about the interactions between societal reactions to homosexual lifestyles in these countries and STD rates? We are thus looking for the common variables as well as the more subtle interplay between culture and illness. Finally, this chapter looks at some of other implicated social and psychological factors in more depth in a replication study. The use of two studies, the first one in four different countries, provides the opportunity not only for investigation of social and cultural variables associated with STDs but also for replication and an assessment of the general supracultural forces operating. As a consequence, we can be reasonably certain that the epidemiological pointers derived from this chapter are neither statistical artifact nor culture-bound.

PSYCHOLOGICAL CORRELATES OF NUMBER OF STD INFECTIONS IN SWEDEN, AUSTRALIA, FINLAND, AND IRELAND

Psychosocial predictors of number of STD infections in homosexual men in four Western countries have been analyzed using three levels: never infected, once infected, and infected two or more times. Given the chance element in STD infection, or for that matter any infection, it is debatable whether the category of one infected reflects a greater risk than never infected or a chance occurrence. On the other hand, the use of three categories provides an opportunity to evaluate whether significant differences are linear or nonlinear: it will become apparent that some of the nonlinear relationships between STDs and social and psychological variables are of considerable interest.

Sweden

Those variables in which there was a significant difference between at least two of the three groups using the least-squares difference criterion at the 10 percent level on one-way analysis of variance are shown on Table 5.1.

The first set of variables that differentiate the three groups, both in a linear fashion, is the temporal variables. Both the age at which respondents became homosexually active and the time elapsed since becoming homosexually active indicated that the multiple infectees (the 2+ group) had become homosexually active earlier than, and had been active longer than, the single infectees, who in turn had a longer time sexually active than those never infected. This suggests that a mechanistic temporal variable may be operating in that the longer an individual has been homosexually active, the higher the chance of becoming infected by chance. On the other hand, it may also be the case that those who start their homosexual activity earliest are more prone to contracting STDs, possibly because their formative homosexual experience occurred at a period where there is usually more emphasis on sexual contact rather than sexual relationships.

A second variable that discriminates the three groups in a linear fashion is masculinity as measured by the Bem Sex Role Inventory (BSRI). Multiple infectees are significantly more "masculine" than single infectees who are significantly more masculine than those never infected. In this case, "masculinity" refers to instrumental behavior, with individuals scoring high on the scale be described as more inde-

TABLE 5.1 Significant Relationships between Social and Psychological
Factors and Number of Sexually Transmitted Disease Infections in Swedish
Homosexual Men

	Times Infected		
	0(53%)	1(17%)	2+(30%)
Actual societal reaction against homosexuality	30.2	34.3*	30.1
Masculinity	2.1	2.3	2.5*
Influence of father on behavior[a]	3.7	4.3	4.4*
Influence of female peers on behavior[a]	5.5*	5.5	4.9
Age at which became homosexually active	21.8*	21.8	19.8
Time elapsed since becoming homosexually active	8.8	10.4	10.9*
% leisure time spent in homosexual subculture when first became homosexually active[a]	55.4	58.0	63.0*
Social class:			
Upper	11	21	31*
Middle	54	45	38
Working	35	34	31
Ever had homosexual relationships more than 2 years:			
Yes	39	59	55*
No	61	41	45
Self-description:[a]			
Sexy	4.2	4.0	3.5*
Clean-shaven	4.4*	3.9	3.5
Extroverted	5.8	6.0	6.4*
Rugged	2.0	2.6	2.6
Preferred partner:[a]			
Passive	3.5	3.4	2.9*
Extroverted	6.3*	6.9	6.9*
Unintelligent	3.1	2.8	2.4*
Socially involved	4.5	3.6*	4.2
Warm	5.6	6.0*	5.7
Well-dressed	4.3	3.8	3.3*
Rugged	2.5	2.6	3.2*
Similar interests	4.0*	4.7	4.8

[a] 0-8 scale.
*$p < .1$

pendent, forceful, dominant, aggressive, acting as a
leader, and having a strong personality. Such individuals
are typical of the male stereotype for whom number of
sexual conquests is an index of masculinity, and it is not
surprising that this is such a strong correlate of number of
STD infections. An interesting parallel to this is the

influence of the father on behavior: again, in a linear fashion, the father (a masculine role model) had a greater influence on those infected compared with those never infected, reinforcing the argument that masculine role and behavior is an important precursor of STD infection. Of further interest is the finding that female peers had less influence on those with multiple infections, which further reinforces the role model hypothesis.

Similarly, the measure of degree of socialization into the homosexual subculture, percentage of leisure time spent in the subculture when the individual first became homosexually active, shows that a similar pattern exists; this tends to support the hypothesis that formative experiences at the time of becoming homosexually active may influence later STD history. However, a nonlinear relationship with STD infections does occur with the actual reaction experienced by homosexual men to their homosexuality by significant others (actual societal reaction against homosexuality). It is difficult to interpret the elevated negative reaction in the single infection group, except to tentatively suggest that in a society where homosexuality is accepted probably as much as in any other Western society, individuals with both high and low levels of sexual interaction appear to have been accepted by their significant others and thus possibly have no need to overcompensate for rejection by increasing sexual interactions or at the high level to decrease due to societal pressure.

Two other variables also relate to number of STD infections: social class and previous relationships. There is a disproportionately high number of respondents who label themselves as "upper class" who have high numbers of infections, and the reverse occurring with those who label themselves as "middle class." It is possible that this is a function again of role models in Swedish society, with middle class models being more staid than upper socioeconomic levels in which there may be fewer social restraints. Of interest also is the fact that significantly more of those with higher numbers of infections have had a previous homosexual relationship lasting more than two years. This effectively negates the argument that those with more STD infections are less capable of forming relationships.

Self-description of the Swedish homosexual men also revealed some interesting differences between the three groups. Compared with those infected once or never, the multiple infectees described themselves to be less sexy, less often clean-shaven, more extroverted, and more rugged. These self-descriptors all reinforce the masculine image, suggesting strongly that the masculine role is an integral part of risk factors. The belief that multiple infectees are *less* sexy than the two other groups does contain the implication that there may be an attempt to compensate for this.

Preferred partner characteristics may also give useful clues to the epidemiology of STDs, since the partner is the other side of the equation. In the preferred partner characteristics that significantly differentiate those with multiple, one, and no STD infections, two points are of particular interest: first, that many of the attributes chosen also reflect dimensions of "masculinity," such as rugged, passive, extroverted. Second, they are all in the same direction as the self-descriptors of the multiple-infected group, suggesting that high-risk factors include a preference for like partners. This would have the effect of multiplication of risk factors, and may partly explain why the Swedish group has the highest proportion of people with one or more STD infections of the four countries studied. Interestingly, Ross (1985d) found that in these four societies, in the more sex-role liberal and less antihomosexual (Sweden), homosexual men preferred like partners rather than opposites; the reverse held for the more sex-role rigid and most antihomosexual. It is thus not surprising to find the multiple-infection group most preferring partners with similar interests, and less well-dressed and more intelligent compared in a linear fashion with the other two groups; both of these dimensions can easily be related to masculinity.

There is no obvious reason why single infectees should prefer more warm and less socially involved partners, but the self-descriptors and preferred partner descriptors in the Swedish sample do reinforce two points of interest in the epidemiology of STD infections: there does appear to be an element of masculine sex role in the risk factors, and there is some strong evidence that partner preferences may emerge as an important variable worth further critical examination at a later stage.

Australia

The same procedure used for the Swedish sample was also adopted for the Australian one: variables that differentiated between the three groups (never infected, once infected, and multiple STD infections) at below the 10 percent level of significance were included for discussion. These results appear in Table 5.2.

Again, as in the Swedish sample, temporal variables appear several times, reinforcing the argument that there is

TABLE 5.2 Significant Relationships between Social and Psychological Factors and Number of Sexually Transmitted Disease Infections in Australian Homosexual Men

	Times Infected		
	0(63%)	1(12%)	2+(25%)
Age	30.6	32.4	35.1*
Kinsey Scale position	5.5	4.8*	5.4
Actual societal reaction against homosexuality	35.2	27.6*	38.5
Influence of father on behavior[a]	3.4	2.9	2.2*
Influence of female peers on behavior[a]	2.6	1.8	1.7*
Age at which realized was homosexual	13.2	16.6*	14.6
Time elapsed since becoming homosexually active	11.0	11.6	16.7
Time elapsed between realizing homosexuality and becoming homosexually active	6.4	4.2	3.8*
% leisure time spent in homosexual subculture and becoming homosexually active	63.8	61.1	51.0*
% leisure time spent in homosexual subculture now	63.1	65.8	70.1*
Self-description:[a]			
Not emotional	3.6	4.4*	3.8
Conventional	5.2	5.9*	4.9
Passive	4.4	3.7*	4.6
Extroverted	4.7	4.9	5.5*
Socially involved	3.6*	4.3	4.2
Clean-shaven	4.4	3.2*	4.3
Large penis	3.3	4.2*	3.5
Preferred partner:[a]			
Not emotional	3.8	4.0	4.3*
Sexy	4.7	5.1*	4.3
Passive	3.8	4.9*	4.5
Unintelligent	2.8*	3.2	3.2
Tall	3.8	3.8	4.4*
Large penis	3.5	4.0	4.1*
Rugged	4.5	3.8	4.6

[a]0-8 scale.

*$p < .1$

a significant degree of chance in whether individuals contract an STD. Four temporal variables significantly differentiated the three levels of infection groups: age, age at which respondents realized they were homosexual, time elapsed since becoming homosexually active, and the time between respondents realizing they were homosexual and becoming homosexually active. In all cases with the exception of age at which individuals realized they were homosexual, the results follow the same linear pattern with the multiple infection group having more time to become infected compared with the once-infected group, who were in turn higher than the never-infected group. The pattern is identical with that in the Swedish data and thus rein-forces the arguments raised that both chance, and appar-ently a more rapid coming out, characterize the higher-risk groups.

Compared with the Swedish sample, the higher-risk group were significantly less socialized into the homosexual subculture when they first became homosexually active, but at the time of data collection were more involved in the homosexual subculture. This last finding does suggest that those at higher risk have both more involvement in places where partners are more available and probably a greater investment in their sexual lifestyle.

It is difficult to interpret the finding that the single infection group is significantly more heterosexual than the other two groups, but the presence of the same two vari-ables of influence on behavior of father and female peers as in the Swedish sample is revealing. However, the direction is reversed in that the father has *less* influence on behav-ior for the multiple infectees, although the influence of female peers is, as in the Swedish sample, lowest in the multiple-infection group. It may be that the influence of the father interacts with the sex-role rigidity of the society, and thus in Australia where male-female roles are more rigid and society more antihomosexual these mitigate against the father being seen as an appropriate model. Actual reaction to homosexuality by significant others also reverses the Swedish pattern.

Self-descriptions that differentiate the three groups of infections are in the case of extroversion identical to the Swedish sample, but beyond this there are major differ-ences. The pattern in the Australian sample is a nonlinear one, with the once-infected or middle-risk group being described as less emotional, more conventional, less pas-sive, less often clean-shaven, and more often having a large penis. While the dimensions are, as in the Swedish data, clearly masculinity related, it is difficult to speculate as to why both high-risk and low-risk groups are low on these variables, unless we speculate that the high-risk group are a subset of the less assertive ("masculine") who attempt to compensate by increasing either particular sexual practices or partner numbers.

Preferred partner characteristics also follow the same nonlinear pattern, suggesting that this is not simply due to chance but has some meaning. Again, the single infection group preferred partners who were more sexy and most passive and least rugged, suggesting the preference of *unlike* partners. This again is consistent with the finding of Ross (1985d) that in the more sex-role rigid and anti-homosexual societies, preferred partners are more likely to be dissimilar on most dimensions on which they may be described. On the other hand, the high-risk group of multiple infectees did prefer the most unemotional, unintelligent, tall, and well-endowed partners, suggesting a preference for lack of psychological involvement with, and emphasis on physical characteristics of, partners is associated with a higher risk. Thus far, it is particularly interesting to note that there are a number of consistencies emerging across societies as well as culture-specific manifestations.

Finland

Again, the groups used and levels of significance are identical to those used in the two preceding groups: data are presented in Table 5.3 for Finnish homosexual men. Parallels between the data for Finland and for Sweden and Australia are striking, with temporal variables again emphasizing the fact that the highest risk group became homosexually active earliest and become homosexually active soonest after realizing they were homosexual. These data reinforce the argument raised earlier that those at highest risk for STD infection are those with the least doubt about their sexual orientation (and perhaps more impulsive in making their sexual contacts) and those whose sexual socialization into a homosexual lifestyle occurs at a point where sexual interactions are of more interest than psychological ones. Similarly, the Finnish data do suggest that those at highest risk spend more time in the homosexual subculture and presumably that they have more investment in their homosexuality than those at lower risk.

As is also the case in the previous data, there is confirmation that those who have had a previous homosexual relationship for more than two years are more likely to have contracted an STD and there is also less influence of female peers on behavior in the higher-risk groups. This last point again suggests that sexual socialization may be an important variable for future research. Years of education does differentiate the three groups, but in a nonlinear fashion, and as a consequence is difficult to interpret.

Self-description of those at higher risk reveals that those with multiple infections see themselves as less emo-

TABLE 5.3 Significant Relationships between Social and Psychological
Factors and Number of Sexually Transmitted Disease Infections in Finnish
Homosexual Men

	Times Infected		
	0(67%)	1(23%)	2+(10%)
Years of education	11.9	13.7*	11.3
Age became actively homosexual	20.4	21.5	18.4*
Time between realizing homosexuality and becoming homosexually active	5.6	7.8*	4.1
% leisure time spent in homosexual subculture now	56.1	58.9	61.4*
Ever had homosexual relationship more than 2 years			
Yes	38	55	54
No	62	45	46
Influence of female peers on behavior[a]	3.1	2.2	2.2*
Self-description:[a]			
Emotional	4.7	4.6	3.3*
Extroverted	5.7	6.1	6.9*
Socially involved	3.4	4.0	5.1*
Short hair	5.8	6.3	6.6*
Rugged	0.8	1.4	1.6*
Preferred partner:[a]			
Passive	3.1	3.4	3.9*
Socially involved	4.1	4.2	5.2*
Feminine	3.2	3.7	4.0*
Short hair	5.8	6.4	6.9*
Similar interests	4.7	4.6	4.0*

[a]0-8 scale.
*$p < .1$

tional, more extroverted, and socially involved, having
shorter hair and being more rugged: again, we see individuals who fit a masculine stereotype and are most likely
to have the social ability to make sexual contacts. Preferred partners are, interestingly, dissimilar in that they
are likely to be more passive and feminine and less likely to
have similar interests. Given that Finland has the lowest
rate of STD infection of the four countries studied, it
appears that partner preferences (similar or dissimilar) may
be one of the more important variables in determining levels
of STD infection to emerge from this analysis.

In general, then, there are already clear cross-cultural
trends emerging from the three societies so far examined.

In many ways the data for the Irish sample will help to support or disconfirm the trends already noted.

Ireland

As with the previous three samples, the Irish sample was divided into three groups (never infected, once infected, and multiple STD infections) and those variables that discriminated between one or more groups at a 10 percent level of significance or lower were retained for analysis. They appear in Table 5.4.

It is of great interest that many of the variables previously implicated in high risk of STD infection have again appeared and been implicated in the Irish sample. Masculinity as measured by the BSRI has again discriminated between the three groups, with the more "masculine" having more STD infections. The multiple infection group similarly became homosexually active earlier, and spends more leisure time in the homosexual subculture, confirming that psychological investment in a homosexual lifestyle and early socialization are cross-culturally common correlates of a high number of STD infections. As in the Finnish sample, education level was highest for the once-infected, suggesting that the better educated are less likely to fall to either extreme of no or multiple STD infections. Similarly, the majority of the multiple infection group had been in a homosexual relationship for longer than two years, as in the Finnish and Swedish samples.

Influences on behavior reveal an unusal pattern: the highest risk group reports that teachers and school had a stronger influence on their behavior than the two lower risk groups, and the single infection group report that they got on significantly worse with their mothers in adolescence: this pattern does not correspond with that in any of the other samples. On the other hand, self-descriptions follow a pattern similar to that of the Australian sample, in which the once-infected group describe themselves as less intelligent, more feminine, less rugged, and more passive. The only exception to this nonlinear trend was the tendency of the multiple infection group to see themselves as more sexy. Again, the adjectives reflect dimensions of masculine sex role, although the pattern is not linear in terms of risk.

Partner preference also tends to reflect masculine sex role attributes, with preferred partners being more sexy, more passive, less intelligent, more clean-shaven, and having more dissimilar interests, while being less conventional. As with the Finnish sample, more dissimilar

TABLE 5.4 Significant Relationships between Social and Psychological Factors and Number of Sexually Transmitted Disease Infections in Irish Homosexual Men

	Times Infected		
	0(63%)	1(12%)	2+(20%)
Years of education	12.9	15.7*	14.1
Masculinity	2.0	2.2	2.6*
How well got on with mother up to adolescence[a]	5.4	4.0*	5.3
Influence of teachers and school on behavior[a]	2.3	2.3	3.7*
Age became homosexually active	21.8	19.5	18.9*
% leisure time spent in homosexual subculture	59.5	64.1	71.4*
Ever had homosexual relationship more than 2 years			
Yes	32	20	63
No	68	80	37
Self-description:[a]			
Sexy	4.0	4.0	4.9*
Passive	4.3	5.3*	3.5
Unintelligent	2.7	3.4*	2.5
Feminine	3.2	3.8*	2.9
Rugged	3.4	2.2*	3.5
Preferred partner:[a]			
Conventional	5.5	4.7	4.0
Sexy	4.7	5.1	5.4*
Passive	4.1	3.8	3.3*
Unintelligent	2.9*	2.6	2.4
Clean-shaven	3.1	4.8	4.9
Similar interests	4.9	3.9	3.6

[a]0-8 scale.
*$p < .1$

partners are preferred by the highest risk group, and again this may have some implications for level of STD infection in these two countries, which are the two lowest of the four countries sampled.

In general, however, the degree of similarity between the four countries is surprising, and what clearly emerge as having epidemiological significance are masculine sex role, extroversion, and social involvement, temporal variables such as the amount of time within which it was possible to contract an STD, early involvement in homosexual activity and socialization into a homosexual model, relationship with father, and similarity or dissimilarity of preferred partner to self. It is therefore of interest to look at the same analysis combining the four samples together in order to look at any general trends that emerge across cultures that have not been picked up in previous analyses.

COMBINED SAMPLES COMPARISONS

On combining the samples from Sweden, Australia, Finland, and Ireland together, and collapsing the three infection level groups into two, never infected (62 percent) and ever infected (38 percent) and comparing the variables on two-tailed t test or χ^2 test, a general view of the variables broadly differentiating those never and ever infected can be gained independent of cultural influences.

The predictors, described below in order of level of significance, were similar to those found within each country. Variables discriminating at beyond the 1 percent level included the following:

- masculinity (infected respondents more "masculine")
- time since became actively homosexual (infected respondents longer)
- social class (infected respondents more often described background as "upper")
- number of partners in past year (infected respondents higher)
- anal-insertor role in sex (infected more often insertors)
- sadomasochistic practices (infected practiced these more often)
- belief that the laws in one's country were prohomosexual (infected believed them to be more prohomosexual)
- proportion of leisure time spent in homosexual subculture (infected respondents higher)

In these predictors at a high level of statistical significance are temporal variables, masculine sex role and instrumental, controlling behavior, particular sexual practices and partner numbers that are congruent with such behavior, social class variables that suggest less socialization into middle-class sexual mores, investment and involvement in the homosexual subculture, and interestingly the belief that one is in a prohomosexual environment, which presumably acts as a disinhibitor or justifier of homosexual behavior.

Those variables that discriminate between the two groups at between the 1 percent and 5 percent levels of significance include the following:

- age (infected respondents older)
- belief that the people in one's country were prohomo-sexual (infected respondents believe them to be more prohomosexual)
- self-rating as clean-shaven (infected respondents less often)
- self-rating as having small penis (infected respondents more often)
- time between realizing was homosexual and becoming actively homosexual (infected respondents shorter time)

Variables that discriminated the two groups at between the 5 percent and 10 percent levels included the following:

- influence of female peers on behavior (infected respondents lower)
- self-rating as extroverted (infected respondents higher)
- preferred partner rating as passive (infected respondents higher)
- preferred partner rating as rugged (infected respondents lower)
- age became actively homosexual (infected earlier)
- heterosexual relationship more than 2 years (infected respondents more often yes)
- anal intercourse, both insertor and insertee (infected respondents higher)

These variables again confirm the trends found in the four-country analyses separately; and these variables also include again sexual practices, partner variables, and self-rated variables all related to masculine response style, earlier socialization into and commencement of homosexual activity, less influence of female peer models (which is possibly related to masculine sex role and lack of influence of the romantic attachment model), and more frequent bisexual involvement. These data summarize effectively the univariate findings: however, there is probably a great deal of overlap, and as a consequence it is necessary to carry out multiple linear regressions on variables in each country to determine which are the major predictors that subsume the minor ones.

Regression Analysis

In order to decrease the number of variables, regression analyses were carried out. Data were analyzed separately

for each country. Multiple linear regressions were performed on the data with forward inclusion criteria of
p = .15 on the basis of the exploratory nature of the data.
Variables included were those described in the questionnaire, with the dependent variable being the total number
of infections for syphilis, gonorrhea, or any other STD,
combined.

From Table 5.5 it can be seen that between four and
seven variable significantly predicted the number of times
men in each country were infected. These variables were
able to predict between 18.7 percent (Finland) and 41.9
percent (Ireland) of the variance of times infected, a fairly
major proportion considering that social and psychological
factors were being investigated. Seven of the variables
predicted infections in more than one country.

Of particular interest are those variables that were
common to more than one country: sex role (masculinity and
femininity), sex role conservatism, religious commitment,
time since the respondent became homosexually active, the
amount of leisure time spent in the homosexual subculture,
and relationship with the father. In all countries all
variables except sex role conservatism related in the same
direction. Masculinity as measured on the BSRI (defined as
a dominant, controlling personality) was associated with
more infections, and femininity (defined as a passive,
unassertive personality) with fewer infections. Sex role
conservatism was associated with a higher rate of infection
in Finland and a lower one in Australia. This measured the
degree to which respondents felt that women and men would
have equality in a number of areas, and in Finland this was
associated with a higher rate of infection through increased
masculine and assertive behavior, whereas in Australia the
more feminine homosexual men had higher infection rates.
Greater religious commitment in each case led to lower
infection rates, which confirms findings in previous
research. Also in line with previous findings was the fact
that both the length of time since becoming homosexually
active (and hence a longer time in which STD might have
been contracted) and the amount of time spent in the
homosexual subculture (probably reflecting involvement in
the subculture and the importance of a homosexual identity
to the individual) were associated with increased infection
rates.

The association of the relationship with the father and
number of time infected is also of interest. These data
indicated that a bad relationship with the father was likely
to lead to more infections. The psychodynamic implications
are interesting, and might show an attempt to come to terms

TABLE 5.5 Predictors of Infection in Homosexual Men in Four Countries

	B	Beta	Cumulative R^2
Sweden			
Masculinity	0.225	0.452	0.141***
Expected social reaction to homosexuality	0.007	0.300	0.210***
Time since became homosexually active	0.125	0.289	0.282***
Femininity	-0.156	-0.220	0.319***
Social class	-0.796	-0.189	0.350**
Age became homosexually active	-0.086	-0.157	0.371*
Actual social reaction to homosexuality	0.004	0.147	0.391*
Australia			
Femininity	-0.129	-0.247	0.054***
Time since became homosexually active	0.079	0.322	0.103***
Sex role conservatism	-0.054	0.319	0.176***
Religious commitment	0.478	0.178	0.207**
Time spent in homosexual subculture	0.239	0.158	0.234*
Relationship with father	-0.136	-0.152	0.254*
Finland			
Time since became homosexually active	0.063	0.443	0.054***
Age realized was homosexual	0.052	0.341	0.120***
Sex role conservatism	0.025	0.258	0.162***
Religious commitment	0.333	0.169	0.187*
Ireland			
Homosexual relationship more than 2 years	-1.311	-0.454	0.120***
Time spent in homosexual subculture	0.463	0.465	0.251***
Relationship with father	-0.208	-0.309	0.302***
Femininity	-0.064	-0.235	0.353***
Attitudes toward homosexuality	-0.037	-0.206	0.386**
Position on Kinsey Scale	-0.355	-0.188	0.419**

*p < 0.1
**p < 0.05
***p < 0.01

with paternal rejection by making increasing numbers of male sexual contacts to achieve acceptance by other men. At this stage, however, this interpretation is tentative and will clearly require further research.

The variables that were not significantly associated with increased infection were: age, education, and degree of openness about homosexuality. A number of other variables were associated with rate of infection in one country but not others, including expected and actual societal reactions to homosexuality, the age at which the man realized he was homosexual, degree of homosexuality, attitudes to homosexuality, and (particularly in Ireland) whether the man had been in a homosexual relationship for two years or more.

The high degree of similarity between the study populations does implicate psychological factors as well as more mechanical relations to infection with STD, such as time spend in the homosexual subculture and length of time since becoming homosexually active. The pervasiveness of predictive variables such as social sex role, sex role conservatism, and relationship with father, all confirm that the psychological dimension of STD infection in homosexual men may be at least as important as demographic variables, if not more so. Whether such psychological factors operate by increasing numbers of partners or the type of partner who is most likely to be infected is not clear. Number of partners was not a major variable, which suggests that STD infection in homosexual men is *not* simply related to number of partners as a risk factor.

Clearly, the major variables worth further investigation include sex roles, investment in homosexual lifestyle, parental relations and early socialization, and these must feature in future studies of predictors.

SOUTH AUSTRALIAN SAMPLE

The South Australian sample was taken at a time some six years later than the earlier four-country comparison and as part of a research project into AIDS: as a result, the questions asked were different in type and emphasis compared with the earlier study. Nevertheless, it does give an opportunity to test some additional hypotheses regarding the epidemiology of social and psychological factors in STDs: the variables differentiating the three groups were as previously tested (no infection, one infection, and multiple STD infections) but referring to infection over the past year only. Data in Table 5.6 represent those variables that differentiated between at least two of the groups using a least-squares difference criterion after one-way analysis of variance at less than 10 percent probability.

As in previous analyses, proportion of leisure time spent in the homosexual subculture significantly differentiated the groups in a linear fashion as in previous

TABLE 5.6 Significant Relationships between Social and Psychological Factors and Number of Sexually Transmitted Disease Infections in South Australian Homosexual Men

	Times Infected		
	0(69%)	1(18%)	2+(13%)
Sexual activity of 5-point Kinsey-type scale, past year	4.6	4.6	4.0*
% leisure time spent in homosexual subculture	38.5	46.3	52.1
Oral sex[a]	5.3	6.6	6.6
Mutual masturbation[a]	4.5	4.1	3.0
Analingus-passive[a]	1.5	1.7	2.8
Alcohol day per week, past five years	2.6	2.5	1.6
Alcohol drinks per day, past year	2.1	2.5	3.3
Marijuana past year	1.8	3.5*	2.6
Nitrites past five years	1.7	2.5*	0.8
Anxiety past three months[a]	4.2*	3.4	3.4
Depression past three months[a]	2.2*	2.7	3.5*
Parental rearing patterns:			
Mother abusive	8.6	9.6*	8.4
Father depriving	10.6	10.6	8.8*
Mother depriving	10.2	10.4*	9.1
Mother rejecting	13.7	12.8*	15.0
Father overinvolved	14.5*	13.9	12.5
Father tolerant	17.8*	17.3	16.3
Mother tolerant	18.5*	16.9	16.7
Father affectionate	11.4	11.4	9.8*
Mother affectionate	12.3	11.0*	13.4
Father performance-oriented	12.3	11.3*	13.1
Father stimulating	12.0	10.7	9.2*
Mother stimulating	12.0	12.6*	11.2
TA	19.8	16.9*	18.9
Masculinity	10.3	10.6	12.6*
Femininity	18.0*	15.6	14.2
Self-esteem	37.7	40.2*	36.8

[a]0-8 scale.
*p < .1

analyses. Sexual activities also differentiated groups, with those with multiple infections having been more heterosexual in the past year, performed oral sex and passive analingus more frequently than low-risk groups, but mutual masturbation was more common in those at low risk.

With regard to drug use, high-risk group members had alcohol less days per week than low-risk group members in a linear trend, but in terms of drinks per day, the trend was reversed. It would appear that those with multiple infections drink less often but when they do drink, drink a great amount more: this would appear to be consistent with less control being exercised by high-risk group members. For marijuana and volatile nitrites, the higher use was in the one infection group and not easy to interpret: however, it is clear that alcohol follows a pattern different from than of marijuana and nitrites.

Of particular interest are the findings that the no-infection group were significantly more anxious than those with one or more infections, but that this linear trend was reversed for depression, where the multiple infection group was significantly more depressed than the other two groups. It is quite likely that anxiety prevents some individuals from having high numbers of sexual partners, and that higher partner numbers may be part of an attempt to control depression.

Parental rearing patterns are clearly implicated in STD infections from these data. Members of the multiple-infection group describe their fathers as being less depriving, less overinvolved, less tolerant, less affectionate, and less stimulating than those with no infections or one infection, in almost all cases in a linear pattern. It appears clear that those who have the highest number of STD infections also have the most distant and uninvolved fathers. Data on relationship with the mother are less consistent: with the exception that mothers of multiple-infection group members are less tolerant, the pattern is nonlinear and it is the mothers of the one-infection group who are most depriving, rejecting, unaffectionate, and stimulating. These data suggest that negative maternal attitudes to the child during rearing have a less strong and less consistent effect than negative paternal attitudes but that they nevertheless constitute a risk factor. By contrast, those in a low-risk group have the most positive paternal and maternal attitudes shown to them by their parents. These data are sufficiently consistent to require follow-up as a psychological factor of some importance in the epidemiology of STDs.

Four other variables of some potential importance emerge. Looking at mood state as measured by the Profile of Mood States the no-infection group is highest on tension-anxiety, the single infection group lowest. Of particular interest is that self-esteem, a possible intervening variable between partner numbers and number of STDs, is an inverted U-shape, with the single infection group having the highest self-esteem (as measured by the Rosenberg scale), the multiple infection group the lowest. These figures certainly support the hypothesis that self-esteem may be an intervening variable of some importance since they are consistent with expectations and the anxiety and depression scale scores.

Finally, the masculinity and femininity scores as measured on the BSRI are entirely consistent with the findings described above in the four-country study.

CONCLUSIONS

The data from two different case-control studies of four different countries provide ample evidence for the existence of social and psychological correlates of levels of STD infection in homosexual men. Those variables implicated across cultures include masculine sex role, early socialization into the homosexual subculture, time spend actively homosexual, parental rearing patterns and relationships, self-esteem, anxiety and depression, investment in homosexuality, sexual practices, education and class, and previous history of relationships. Those implicated within cultures include particularly preferred partner characteristics and their interactions with self-perception and the sex-role rigidity and antihomosexual attitudes of the country.

Given that there are a number of consistent and coherent epidemiological patterns that emerge from these studies, it is necessary to determine which of the particular variables may directly influence whether an individual contracts an STD and how frequently. These variables include partner numbers, sexual activities, partner characteristics and possibly setting of partner contact, and chance and temporal variables. With the exception of chance and temporal variables, the following chapters examine these variables in detail in an attempt to describe how they influence STD infection and whether increased understanding may lead to possible interventions.

6

Partner Numbers in Homosexual Men: A Psychosocial Analysis

Schofield (1976) comments that "to describe promiscuity as a sickness is to use the term to disguise moral disapproval. It is part of the unfortunate tendency to regard a man as sick because he does not conform." Today, while we would also regard the word "promiscuity" as implying moral disapproval (and it is used in this chapter only as it has been used by those cited), the basic hypotheses as to why individuals have high numbers of partners have remained. In most discussions of the precursors of STD infection, high partner numbers are listed and the suggestion made that such individuals who are "promiscuous" are maladjusted. On the other hand, Schofield has suggested that increased partner numbers are also the result of hedonism, and that (in his study of heterosexuals in 1976) there was little if any evidence that those with high partner numbers have personality defects, are emotionally damaged, or came from a less than adequate social milieu. On the contrary, he found that those with higher partner numbers were better educated, and that "promiscuity" was a factor in only half of the cases of STD infection he studied. Thus, while most individuals associate partner numbers with STD infections, the association is neither a clear-cut nor a necessary or sufficient one.

Little work has been carried out on the associations of partner number in homosexual men. Goode and Troiden (1980) looked at promiscuity as a dimension and as a style of sexual expression among homosexual men in several cities in the United States. They found that one-third of the least promiscuous, as compared with two-thirds of the most promiscuous, had had at least one STD, and that the most promiscuous appeared to prefer emotionally superficial sex and tended to have sex only once with more than half their partners as compared with about a quarter of the time in the least promiscuous. Relationships between promiscuity and other variables also suggested that older respondents had contracted more STDs than younger respondents, and that level of education and partner number negatively correlated.

Apart from this study, however, there have been few attempts to investigate the psychosocial correlates of partner numbers in homosexuals, particularly with regard to STDs. The emergence of AIDS in homosexual men with many partners has also increased the clinical significance of gaining an adequate understanding of the relationships between psychosocial variables and high partner numbers; in this context, it is reasonable to speculate that the former may explain a significant proportion of the variance of the latter. In this chapter, therefore, we look at the psychological, social, and demographic variables that are associated with high and low partner numbers in an attempt to establish whether any pattern emerges that may have clinical significance in the modification of this behavior.

PARTNER NUMBERS AND THEIR COVARIATES ACROSS CULTURES

Looking at the associations with partner numbers in the four countries serves two purposes: it allows us to look at the effects of societal and cultural factors on partner numbers, and also to look at variables which are common across cultures. Such analyses, looking at groups of individuals, can only reveal common trends within and between groups, and are unable to reveal separate subgroups, for example, of those with low partner numbers where opposing trends may cancel each other out. The analyses of the four countries (Sweden, Australia, Finland, and Ireland) is based on t test between two groups, those with nil or one partner per month on average, versus those with multiple partners per month. Where variables are discontinuous, the χ^2 test is used. Results are displayed in Table 6.1. It is of interest that the proportions of individuals across the four countries differ significantly, with Sweden and Australia highest and Finland and Ireland lowest. This difference does suggest that cultural factors are operating as determinants of partner numbers, the most

TABLE 6.1 Significant Associations with High Partner Number in Homosexual Men in Four Countries

Variable	Sweden	Austra-lia	Fin-land	Ire-land
% having more than one partner per month	55	46	31	36
Age	↓	--	--	--
Years education	--	--	↓	--
Time since became homosexually active	--	--	--	↑
Anticipated negative societal reaction to homosexuality	--	↓	--	--
Self-rating as emotional	--	↑	--	--
Preferred partner is unconventional	--	--	↑	--
Self-rating as unconventional	--	--	↑	--
Preferred partner is sexy	--	--	↑	--
Self-rating as socially involved	--	--	--	↑
Preferred partner is masculine	--	--	↑	--
Self-rating as tall	--	--	--	↑
Preferred partner is hairy	↑	--	--	--
Self-rating as clean-shaven	--	↑	--	--
Self-rating as long-haired	↓	--	--	--
Self-rating as having large penis	--	↑	--	--
Preferred partner as well-dressed	--	↓	--	--
Self-rating as rugged	↑	--	--	--
Masculinity	↑	--	--	--
Femininity	↓	--	--	--
Times infected with STD	--	--	↑	↑
How much people in their country are antihomosexual compared to other places	--	--	↓	↓
Knew individual from whom caught STD	--	↑	↑	↑
Would there be problems at work if people found out you are homosexual?	↓	--	--	--
From how many heterosexuals do you try to conceal your homosexuality?	↓	--	--	--
Has (or would) being labeled homosexual bother you?	↓	↓	↓	--
Age at which realized was homosexual	--	↓	--	--
How much do you think homosexuality violates Conventional morality?	--	↓	↓	--
Religious (Christian morality?	--	↓	↓	--
Conformity in general?	--	--	↓	--
How much influence did female friends your own age have on you?	--	--	↑	--
How much influence did teachers or school have on you?	--	--	↓	--

TABLE 6.1 Continued

Variable	Sweden	Austra-lia	Fin-land	Ire-land
Age realized people think homosexuality wrong, deviant, or different?	↓	--.	--	--
Prefer anal-insertor sex role	↓	--	--	--
Prefer full body contact sex role	↓	--	--	↑
Prefer S & M sex role	↑	--	--	--
Prefer fellatio, both insertor and insertee	--	↓	--	--
In homosexual relationship more than 2 years at present	--	↓	--	--
Seen psychiatrist about homosexuality	--	↓	--	↑
Religious involvement	--	--	--	↓
Social class	--	--	--	↑

↑ increase in variable associated with high partner numbers
↓ decrease in variable associated with high partner numbers
-- not significant

probable being size of country and degree of industriali-zation as well as size of the major city. It must be borne in mind that the Swedish and Australian samples were taken in cities of a million or more inhabitants, while the Finnish and Irish samples came from cities of half that size. It is thus possible that size of city is an important variable (as suggested by Darrow et al. 1981) in that it provides a homosexual subculture in which sufficient venues and partners are available for those who have large numbers of partners. Within each country, however, patterns of associations with high partner numbers are apparent.

SWEDEN

Few demographic variables discriminate the Swedish homo-sexual men with high partner numbers apart from the fact that they are significantly younger and realized that homo-sexuality was thought to be deviant, different, or wrong at an earlier age. Self-ratings as being shorter-haired, more rugged, more masculine, and less feminine (as measured by the BSRI) give a picture of a conventionally masculine sex role: such a role often includes an image of the masculine man as a seducer and controller of others. Preferred part-ners are more hairy (a masculine attribute).

Psychological variables that distinguish the individual with high partner numbers include less concealment of, and less concern about the consequences of, being labeled as homosexual. In terms of preferred sexual activities, high partner preference individuals prefer the anal-insertor sex role less, full-body contact less, and sadomasochistic practices more than those with low partner numbers. Generally, then, the high partner number Swedish homosexual is masculine, open about his homosexuality, younger and has a preference for several sexual practices.

AUSTRALIA

No demographic variables discriminated those Australian homosexual men who had multiple partners. Those who had the higher partner numbers anticipated a fairly positive societal reaction to homosexuality, and described themselves as more emotional, more often clean-shaven, and as having large genitals. They also reported preferring partners who were casually dressed: it is difficult to see any consistent pattern in these data. They were less concerned about being labeled homosexual, realized they were homosexual at an earlier age, and believed that homosexuality violated traditional mores less severly than those who reported low partner numbers. Sexual practices preferred were fellatio without preference for position, and they were less likely to be in a homosexual relationship at the time of responding or to have ever seen a psychiatrist about their sexual orientation. Again, the pattern that emerges is of little concern about their sexual orientation and a belief that it is not greatly in conflict with social mores.

FINLAND

The Finnish homosexual men who had reported high partner numbers tended to be less well educated than their peers who had fewer contacts, and to have contracted an STD more often. They also tended to rate themselves as more unconventional and to prefer partners who are unconventional, sexy, and masculine. They saw people in their country as less antihomosexual and were less concerned at being labeled as homosexual, and again saw homosexuality as violating conventional mores less. They also reported that female peers had more influence on them, and teachers less influence, than their peers with a lower number of partners.

IRELAND

Irish homosexual men who had the highest partner numbers had been active homosexually longer, saw themselves as more socially involved, and had had more STD infections than their compatriots with lower numbers of partners. They also were of a higher reported social class more frequently, had more often seen a psychiatrist about their homosexuality, preferred full-body contact as a sexual practice more frequently, and were less religiously involved.

In general, these picture of the homosexual men with higher partner numbers are inconsistent and shed little light on the question of whether there are particular cultural influences on partner numbers. There are inconsistencies in the direction of two variables, preference for full-body contact and a history of having seen a psychiatrist about their orientation, which may reflect cultural differences. However, there is little here to suggest that there is any major within-culture variation with regard to variables associated with increased partner numbers, and it can probably be concluded that such culture-specific contributors do not exist.

COMBINED SAMPLES

On the other hand, reference to Table 6.2 confirms that across the combined samples from the four-country study there are some major and consistent trends. Demographic trends that emerged when the samples were collapsed and separated into three groups (nil, one, and multiple different partners per months on average in the past year) showed that those in the one-partner group were different from the other two groups in that they were better educated, more homosexual, and had been actively homosexual for less time than those with nil or multiple partners. They had also become actively homosexual later than the other two groups and in addition realized they were homosexual at a later age. The single-partner group also felt that homosexuality violated conventional and religious morality and conformity in general less than did the other two groups, and anticipated the most negative response from significant others to their homosexuality. However, it was the no-partner group that had *actually* had the worst reaction, and had realized that homosexuality was stigmatized at the oldest age. These data suggest that in some areas, it is the middle group rather then the two extremes of partner numbers that may be atypical.

TABLE 6.2 Significant Differences between Nil, One, and Multiple Partners per Month and Psychosocial Variables in Four-Country Combined Sample

Variable	0	1	2+
Years education	11.6	13.3*	11.8
Position on Kinsey Scale	5.2	5.4*	5.2
Years actively homosexual	9.5	8.7*	10.5
Actual societal reaction of significant others to homosexuality	3.4*	3.1	3.2
Expected societal reaction of significant others to homosexuality	5.1	5.4*	5.1
Age became actively homosexual	20.7	21.5*	19.7
Age realized was homosexual	14.7	15.8*	14.2
Belief that homosexuality violates:			
Conventional morality	4.6	4.1*	4.8
Religious (Christian) morality	4.3	3.9*	4.4
Conformity in general	4.9	4.5*	5.2
Influence of mother on behavior	4.1	4.4*	4.0
Influence of teachers and school on behavior	4.8	4.8	5.1*
Age when realized people think homosexuality wrong, deviant, or different	14.4*	13.7	13.6
Self-rating:			
Conventional	5.0*	4.6	4.5
Not sexy	4.5	4.4	4.0*
Passive	4.2	4.2	3.9*
Extroverted	5.4	5.5	5.7*
Short	4.4*	4.2	4.0
Not hairy	5.4*	5.3	4.9
Short hair	6.1*	6.0	5.7
Small penis	4.5	4.5	4.0*
Delicate	5.8*	5.6	5.2
Preferred partner:			
Not sexy	3.4	3.3	3.1*
Extroverted	6.6*	6.3	6.3
Not socially involved	3.7	3.9	4.2*
Cold	2.4	2.6*	2.5
Not hairy	5.2	5.3	4.8*
Long hair	6.1*	4.7	4.5
Small penis	3.8	4.1*	3.8
Casually dressed	4.2	4.3	4.6*
Similar interests	3.2*	3.4	3.5
Masculinity	21.6	21.6	22.6*
Times infected with STD	0.4	0.9	1.4*
Extent to which laws in country seen as antihomosexual, compared to other places	4.2	4.3	4.7*
Extent to which people in country seen as antihomosexual, compared to other places	3.8	3.9	4.5*

TABLE 6.2 Continued

Variable	0	1	2+
Sex role conservatism	38.5*	34.3	35.8
How much respondents think significant others would react negatively to their homosexuality:			
Mother	2.5	2.6	2.1*
Brother	2.0	2.0	1.6*
Aunts	3.7	4.4*	3.9
Father	3.0	3.7*	3.0
Sister	1.6	1.9*	1.3
Uncles	4.1	4.5*	3.9
Best same-sex heterosexual friend	1.7*	1.3	1.1
Teachers	3.2	3.2	2.9*
Grandparents	3.5	4.1*	3.6
People at work	3.0	3.5*	2.9
Neighbors	4.1	4.6*	3.5
Customers/clients	2.9	2.9*	2.5
Other same-sex heterosexual friends	2.6	2.9*	2.5
Best opposite-sex heterosexual friend	1.4*	1.2	0.9
Ministers of religion	3.6	4.0*	3.2
Work associates	2.9	3.5*	2.7
Your boss	3.0	3.7*	2.9
Heterosexuals in general	3.8	4.6*	3.6
Friends of parents	4.3	4.9*	3.9
Most opposite-sex heterosexual friends	2.7	2.9*	2.4
How much respondent's significant others have reacted to their homosexuality:			
Aunts	1.0	1.1*	0.8
Best same-sex heterosexual friend	1.3	1.6*	1.5
Teachers	0.8	0.6*	0.9
Grandparents	0.8	0.3*	0.7
People at work	1.3	0.9*	1.4
Neighbors	1.0	0.7*	1.3
Customers/clients	0.8	0.4*	0.8
Sister	1.0	0.8*	1.1
Ministers of religion	1.2	0.6*	1.2
Work associates	1.0	0.8*	1.1
Your boss	1.0	0.7*	1.0
Heterosexuals in general	1.2	0.7*	1.3
Friends of parents	1.0	0.7*	1.1

TABLE 6.2 Continued

Variable	0	1	2+
From how many heterosexuals do you conceal your homosexuality?[a]	2.3	2.3	2.0*
Would there be problems at work if people found out?[a]	0.7	0.7	0.5*
Do you think people are likely to break off a social relationship with someone they think is homosexual?[a]	1.5	1.4	1.3*
Do you think people are likely to make life hard for someone they think is homosexual?[a]	1.4*	1.2	1.2

[a] 0-5 scale.

*$p < .1$

On self-rating, however, there did appear to be a linear rather than curvilinear trend. The multiple partner group rated themselves as less conventional, more sexy, less passive, more extroverted, taller, hairier and with shorter hair, more rugged and with larger genitals than the one-partner group, who were in turn higher than the no-partner group. This relative linearity does suggest that those with higher partner numbers are likely to be correspondingly higher on all of these masculine sex role descriptors. This masculine image, noted earlier as one of the strongest epidemiological correlates of STD infection, is thus strongly implicated through partner numbers as a contributor to STD infection.

Preferred partner characteristics are also, with only a couple of exceptions, linear in their relationship with partner numbers. The respondents with the highest partner numbers preferred sexual contacts who were most sexy, more introverted, more socially involved, and had dissimilar interests. Physically, the respondents with the highest partner numbers preferred sex with men who were hairy, had short hair, and were casually dressed. They were also more masculine as measured by the BSRI, and most likely to see the laws and the people in their country as less anti-homosexual than the other groups. Interestingly, they were less sex-role conservative than the no-partner group.

The fairly consistent linear relationship across the three groups in terms of self-rating and preferred partner characteristics gives way to an entirely different pattern in terms of how negatively individuals thought significant others *would* react if they were told about their homosexual orientation. As can be clearly seen in Table 6.2, with few exceptions it was the single-partner group who were most likely to expect the most negative reaction from significant others: the exceptions were two immediate family members (mother and brother) in whom the multiple-partner group were most likely to expect the most positive reaction (in line with their expectations of people and laws in their country being least antihomosexual).

Looking at the reaction of significant others who *had* reacted to the respondent's homosexuality, the single-partner group was again the group consistently different from the other two groups, in that (with the exception of aunts and best same-sex heterosexual friend) they had received the most positive response to their coming out as a homosexual to these individuals. These data are of particular interest in that they are both discordant in direction and particularly because they suggest that there is a nonlinear relationship between these variables and partner numbers. These data either suggest that the single-partner group are those who most misperceive reactions to themselves, or in direct contrast are most likely to "come out" only to those from whom they expect a positive reaction, and not to "come out" as homosexual to those from whom they expect the most negative reaction. This latter explanation is the most likely, since it can be seen from Table 6.2 that the multiple-partner group are most likely to expect a generally positive reaction (and, presumably, tell most people) as compared with the two groups. The no-partner group, by contrast, expects the most negative reaction socially to their sexual orientation. Thus it would appear that there is in fact a continuum of response to one's own homosexuality that relates to partner numbers: the individuals with multiple partners assume that all reactions will be positive and tend to come out to more people, while those in the single-partner group come out to those who they believe will be most positive and not to those they consider most negative. Those in the no-partner group come out to very few people, and get much the same reaction as the multiple-partner group.

The second important conclusion that can be drawn from these data is that the no-partner and multiple-partner groups, at least in actual and anticipated societal reaction to their sexual orientation, are almost identical, with the single-partner group being the dissimilar one. In terms of process, this does suggest that the psychodynamics for both high and low partner numbers have a common base, and the different dynamics may be operating for those individuals with a moderate number of partners. It is therefore important to look at data that may either confirm or reject this hypothesis with other variables, and this may be done by looking at the second study, the South Australian one.

THE SOUTH AUSTRALIAN STUDY

Data from the South Australian sample appear in Table 6.3. In contrast to the Swedish sample, older age was associated with *more* STD infections, but those respondents who had been homosexually active the longest also had the highest partner numbers. Whether this reflects the changing norms in homosexual subcultures or is related to aging is not apparent. The respondents with the highest partner numbers were also more homosexual as measured on the Kinsey Scale, possibly because of a similar pattern in percentage of leisure time spent in the homosexual subculture. This latter finding is important, since a greater leisure time spent in contact with other homosexuals not only will emphasize the definition of self as "homosexual" (used as a noun rather than as an adjective) and thus to defining most of one's behaviors and attitudes as "homosexual," but also to defining one's identity in terms of sexual behavior. The centrality of the homosexual identity and thus homosexual role is confirmed by sexual behavior with the same sex; this corresponds with Stage Five in the Cass (1979) model of homosexual adjustment. Cass differentiates Stage Five, where the homosexual identity colors the individual's whole existence, with Stage Six, in which the preference for the same-gender sexual partner is only one aspect of the individual's identity and core personality constructs. These data suggest that partner numbers will be higher in those individuals who are at Stage Five, since the same-gender sexual partners will confirm and support the homosexual identity.

Several other pieces of information are congruent with previous findings. Those with higher partner numbers drink alcohol on fewer days per week, but when they do drink, have substantially more to drink than those with nil or one partners. These data strongly suggest that the multiple-partner group are binge drinkers rather than regular social drinkers, and raise the possibility that lack of inhibition or discrimination may in some cases be associated with excessive alcohol consumption. It is particularly

TABLE 6.3 Significant Associations with Nil, One, and Multiple Partners per Month in South Australian Homosexual Men

Variable	0	1	2+
Age	31.8	32.9	36.4*
Kinsey Scale position, past year	5.5	5.8	6.0*
Kinsey Scale position, past 5 years	5.3	5.5	5.9*
% leisure time spent in homosexual subculture	37.5	43.8	48.1*
Analingus-active[a]	1.4	2.3*	1.5
Years homosexually active	10.5	12.2	.18.9
Alcohol days per week past 5 years	3.0*	2.4	1.8
Alcohol drinks per day past year	2.2	2.2	3.2*
Alcohol drinks per day past 5 years	2.1	2.4	3.1*
Stress past 3 months[a]	5.3*	4.5	4.2
Times infected with STD past year	0.3	0.6	0.8*
Times infected with STD past 5 years	1.5	2.3	3.0*
Parental rearing patterns:			
Father abusive	8.5	9.8	9.9*
Father punitive	12.8	14.7*	14.0
Father overprotective	14.5	16.7*	15.6
Father overinvolved	12.8	15.8*	14.1
Father affectionate	11.7*	11.2	10.1
Father guilt-engendering	7.8	8.9*	8.5
Mother depriving	9.6	10.6*	10.3
Mother punitive	12.8	14.5*	12.2
Mother shaming	7.6	8.6*	7.3
Mother overinvolved	14.5	16.5*	16.4
Mother tolerant	18.6*	17.5	17.5
Mother affectionate	12.8	11.7*	12.2
Mother stimulating	12.9	10.8*	12.6
Mother favors siblings	6.4*	7.7	7.7
Mother favors respondent	8.0*	6.8	6.8
Father factor 1 (negative)	38.3	45.4*	45.0
Father factor 3 (favors siblings)	12.3*	14.7*	13.4
Mother factor 2 (positive)	47.4	37.5*	43.8
Mother factor 3 (favors siblings)	8.7*	9.6	9.6
Mood states:			
Confusion	15.0*	13.8	12.7
Fatigue	16.7*	15.7	13.9

[a] 0-8 scale

*$p < .1$

97

interesting that there is no association between use of any other drugs (marijuana, volatile nitrites, or street drugs) and partner levels. On the other hand, many of the places where partners may be met serve alcohol, and it may be that the association between alcohol and partner numbers is a spurious one due to the type of premises at which partners are picked up. As expected, there was also a linear relationship between the number of sexual contacts on average per month in the past year and number of STD infections in the past year and past five years, confirming that number of partners is one of the major risk factors for STD infection.

Parental rearing patterns were looked at in some detail in the South Australian sample, since they were implicated in previous work (Ross 1984d) on partner numbers. The parental rearing history of respondents as measured by the EMBU inventory of parental rearing patterns was used as the most appropriate measure, and the results can be seen in Table 6.3. Of particular interest is the fact that of the 14 scales for each parent, 15 in total were significantly associated with partner numbers. The fact that more than half were associated with partner numbers is a clear indication that parental rearing is an important factor in determining this variable, as has previously been suggested. The contribution of the mother is probably greater, as suggested by the fact that the contribution of the mother as measured by the number of mother-related scales to father-related scales is increased by half.

Looking first at the contribution of the father, it is apparent that the scores on negative rearing patterns are significantly higher for the one-partner and multiple-partner groups than for the no-partner group. Fathers of no-partner men were less abusive, punitive, overprotective, overinvolved, and guilt-engendering, and more affectionate. However, the one-partner group was higher than the multiple-partner group. Interestingly, we see much the same pattern emerging in some of the scales that measure mother's parental rearing patterns. Mothers of the no-partner group were consistently less depriving and less overinvolved, favored the respondent more, and were more tolerant. However, it was the mothers of the one-partner group who were most punitive and shaming, and least affectionate and stimulating. These patterns suggest some particularly interesting dynamics in the genesis of high partner number preference in homosexual men.

First, it would appear that a negative paternal rearing pattern predisposes to higher partner numbers, *but* that within this group (one through to multiple partners), the more negative the pattern, the less the partner numbers. Thus, we are looking at a two-stage set of dynamics that reveals an inverted-U curve with regard to the role of the father, and also with regard to the role of the mother being depriving and overinvolved. Second, a positive maternal rearing pattern (mother not depriving, not overinvolved, and tolerant) will follow the same pattern. Third, however, a mother who is punitive, shaming, unaffectionate and unstimulating will predispose to low partner numbers, *but* within this group (nil or one partner), the more negative, the higher the partner numbers.

Putting these parental dynamics together, it is apparent that the dynamics of the no-partner group are a positive paternal and moderately positive maternal parental rearing pattern; for the multiple-partner group, a positive paternal and a moderately positive maternal rearing pattern are implicated. For the single-partner group, negative paternal and maternal patterns are evidenced. These data, when summarized by looking at factor scores for mother and father on the three major factors extracted from the parental rearing data, suggest that the overall pattern is that positive interactions with father and mother are associated with low partner numbers, and that the most negative parental rearing pattern is associated with a moderate level (for example, one per month) of sexual partners.

In this analysis, then, it appears that the very high and very low levels of partner numbers may have more in common with each other than with the moderate partner level group. While negative experiences predispose to higher partner numbers, the most negative parental rearing pattern tends to decrease the partner numbers within the one-to-multiple partners group. It is of particular interest, therefore, to look at other factors that may covary with parental rearing patterns to influence partner numbers. In Table 6.3, there are three variables that all relate to mood state and external contributors: confusion and fatigue (as measured by the POMS) and stress. In each of these, the pattern is for the highest levels to occur in the no-partner group, and the lowest in the multiple-partner group. It seems fairly clear from these data that dysphoric mood state has the effect of depressing partner numbers, although it could also be interpreted as suggesting that high partner numbers protect against stress, confusion, and fatigue through their effect on increasing self-esteem.

In conclusion, it is apparent that individuals with higher partner numbers differ from those with lower partner numbers on a number of indices. The most consistent of these include parental rearing patterns, stressors, expectations of negative reactions to their homosexuality by significant others and by society in general, masculinity in terms of self-perception and preference for a more feminine partner, and alcohol consumption. The picture that emerges for the high-partner individual is of a male who is conventionally masculine and who believes that there is little negative reaction to his homosexuality. He will have had a more negative parental rearing pattern, and be under less stress than low-partner numbers men, tend to binge-drink alcohol more, be more involved in the homosexual subculture and see his homosexuality as more central to his lifestyle, and have had more STD infections. These data illustrate the multifactorial nature of the variables associated with high partner numbers, ranging from negative parental rearing patterns suggestive of a need to compensate through higher partner numbers, a belief that homosexuality is not perceived negatively by society and by significant others, lack of stressors or dysphoric mood states, and adherence to conventional norms of masculinity including dominance and a perception of the male role as incorporating multiple sexual contracts. This picture is internally consistent across cultures and in the partial replication in South Australia, and suggests that while there is no clear pathology in homosexual men with high or low partner numbers, there are some psychodynamic antecedents that may account for their sexual behavior. On the other hand, the homosexual men with low partner numbers appear to be more concerned about the societal perception of homosexuality and possess a more dysphoric mood state. But it is the homosexual men with moderate partner numbers who emerge as having the most negative relationship with their parents, which suggests that in some ways this group should be looked at separately from the high- and low-partner groups. There are, however, a number of variables that progress in linear fashion through the groups, and these do provide a consistent portrait of the covariates of partner numbers in homosexual men. It is thus fairly clear that there are some strong social, and particularly psychological, associations with partner numbers, including psychodynamic and personality factors: these should be of assistance not only in understanding the at-risk behaviors of homosexual men but also in providing either interventions or health education for this population. Hopefully, an understanding of the dynamics and the more immediate variables that appear to underly variations in partner numbers may help individuals come to terms with factors that may drive them to increased risks through increased partner numbers.

However, these data emphasize that it is impossible to

attribute psychopathology to those with high partner numbers, and that it is equally possible to see negative psychological concommitants in those with low partner numbers or those with moderate partner numbers. These data demonstrate that such attribution of conventional morality to the spectrum of partner numbers is not only unsupported by data but also counterproductive in that it takes no account of what is apparently a complex phenomenon. An understanding of the dynamics of partner numbers of homosexual men does appear possible, but only if it is recognized that many different processes may operate, and that there is no single explanation for what are apparently dissimilar groups in matters other than preference for particular numbers of partners.

7

Sexual Practices and
Their Psychosocial Correlates

Little has been written about the correlates of particular
sexual practices in homosexual men from a psychological
point of view. Indeed, it would appear that the common
assumption is that there are no psychosocial correlates, and
that as a consequence little point in research on this area.
Two stages in the development of this assumption can be
identified: first, that homosexual practices were dependent
on the sex role of the individual, and second, that there
are few preferences for particular activities in homosexual
men.

Initially, it was believed that homosexual men aped
heterosexual relationships, with one playing a "male" and
the other a "female" role. These roles coincided with
insertor and insertee preferences in anal intercourse. Haist
and Hewitt (1974) report that individuals who prefer an
anal-insertee role tend also to prefer an oral-insertee role
in fellatio, and that sex role preferences were consistently
correlated with other sexual and nonsexual behaviors that
can be placed on a masculine-feminine continuum. However,
Hooker (1965) found no relationship between sexual activity
preferences and gender role: it may be that the geographical source of the samples for the two studies account for
this discrepancy, since Haist and Hewitt derived their
samples from the Midwest of the United States, whereas
Hooker's sample was from Southern California.

More recently, it has again been argued that homosexual men rarely have such fixed preferences for sexual

activities, and that sexual activities depend more on the time, place, and participants and cover a wide range of preferences in the one individual. While this belief that sexual activities are polymorphous in the individual is largely correct in the sense that preferences are not strongly held and that as a consequence homosexual men are usually quite willing to vary activity depending on partner, preference at a particular point in time, setting, and so on, there are nevertheless preferences. Insofar as preferences do exist, they have some fairly profound implications for transmission of sexually related diseases.

Most research to date has concentrated on the sexual activity which has been seen to be specific to homosexual men, anal intercourse. In fact, anal intercourse is probably one of the more common contraceptive practices in less developed countries where other forms of contraception are unavailable, but there are few if any studies looking at the incidence of STDs in such populations. However, Bolling (1977) notes that some 8 percent of heterosexual women regularly practice anal receptive intercourse. Activities that are shared with heterosexuals include fellatio, mutual masturbation, full body contact to orgasm (occasionally referred to as frottage, although the term usually refers to clothed bodies), intercrural intercourse, and less commonly, analingus and some sadomasochistic practices.

In terms of the significance of sexual practices for STD transmission, attention has most frequently focused on anorectal sites. There are some good morphological reasons for such a focus, as Ostrow and Altman (1983) point out. Not only is the rectum composed of squamous epithelium as opposed to cornified epithelium in the vagina, but in addition the rectal mucosa is in many places only one cell thick and is thus easily lesioned. This provides a portal of entry for pathogens to a greater extent than would occur vaginally. In addition to this, rectal infection is probably less likely to be noticed than vaginal infection owing to its site, and thus lead to a greater prevalence of asymptomatic infection.

A second risk factor for anorectal sites is exemplified by analingus (oroanal contact). This practice provides an excellent route of transmission for enteric pathogens such as amebiasis, giardiasis, shigellosis, hepatitis, and proctitis due to a number of organisms. Anorectal involvement in sexual practices, whether anal intercourse or analingus, does appear to lead to an increase in hepatitis and the cluster of enteric infections known collectively as "Gay bowel syndrome."

However, there has been little significant work carried

out to determine if there are degrees of preference in
sexual practices, and whether these are related to different
risks. Ross (1985a) found, using discriminant analysis,
that anal sexual practices were associated with an increased
risk of STD infection, and that oral sexual practices were
associated with a decreased risk. Nor has the question as
to whether either degrees of preference, or level of actual
involvement in, particular sexual practices have psychosocial correlates and are thus open to possible modification,
been addressed. This chapter looks at cultural differences
in sexual practices, and then at their associations in terms
of demographic variables, partner preferences, parental
rearing patterns, and attitudes to homosexuality.

FOUR-COUNTRY SAMPLE

Cultural variation in sexual practices, at least as far as
homosexuality is concerned, has been little investigated.
West (1977) has suggested that there may be some differences between homosexual men in Britain and the United
States, with the former appearing to prefer anal intercourse
and the latter fellatio. However, little if any research has
quantified the cultural differences. Table 7.1 illustrates
the differences in preference for sexual activity in homosexual men in Sweden, Finland, Australia, and Ireland who
were asked to check boxes for sexual activities they preferred. Options included fellatio-insertor, fellatio-insertee,
fellatio-both, and anal intercourse-insertor, anal intercourse-insertee, anal intercourse-both, mutual masturbation,
full body contact, and anything else (sadomasochistic practices accounted for 100 percent of this category). Results
appear to support the argument that some cultural differences exist, with four activities showing significantly different trends across samples. Preference for a particular
role in fellatio followed that same pattern for both insertor
and insertee roles, with Swedes preferring the most differentiated roles and the Irish the least. In both cases, the
highest preference is shown in the two larger countries
with the most differentiated homosexual subcultures, suggesting that a greater choice of partners and a more organized homosexual subculture is a determinant of greater
differentiation of sexual activity preferences. On the other
hand, for sexual activities that are equal in terms of role
differentiation, such as mutual masturbation and full body
contact, the Swedes were again the most differentiated, but
the remaining pattern did not reveal any clear evidence as
to why the distribution by country followed the pattern it

TABLE 7.1 Sexual Practice Preferences by Country

	% No Preference	% Prefer
Fellatio-insertor		
Swedes	83.5	16.5
Australians	87.3	12.7
Finns	91.2	8.8
Irish	94.3	5.7*
Fellatio-insertee		
Swedes	84.1	15.9
Australians	91.1	8.9.
Finns	93.9	6.1
Irish	95.1	4.9**
Fellatio-both		
Irish	21.3	78.7
Swedes	30.1	69.9
Australians	30.4	69.6
Finns	32.0	68.0 ns
Anal intercourse-insertor		
Swedes	77.3	22.7
Irish	79.5	20.5
Australians	82.3	17.7
Finns	87.8	12.2 ns
Anal intercourse-insertee		
Swedes	83.0	17.0
Australians	84.2	15.8
Irish	86.9	13.1
Finns	89.1	10.9 ns
Anal intercourse-both		
Finns	53.1	46.9
Swedes	52.3	47.7
Australians	51.9	48.1
Irish	47.5	52.5 ns
Mutual masturbation		
Swedes	32.4	67.6
Finns	44.9	55.1
Australians	56.3	43.7
Irish	56.6	43.4**
Full body contact		
Swedes	12.5	87.5
Irish	19.7	80.3
Australians	25.9	74.1
Finns	29.9	70.1**
Sadomasochistic practices		
Swedes	90.3	9.7
Irish	90.2	9.8
Finns	88.4	11.6
Australians	84.8	15.2 ns

*p < .05; **p < .01

did. While in terms of mutual masturbation the greatest preference occurred in the two sex-role-liberal countries, Sweden and Finland, full body contact did not follow the same pattern. However, it is interesting to note that there were no cultural differences for anal intercourse or sado-masochisitic practices. Given the small sample size for preferences in most practices in each country, however, it was decided to pool the four-country samples in order to examine the common correlates of preference for sexual activities across the samples.

Fellatio

Some remarkably consistent trends across the three fellatio categories are apparent. Table 7.2 illustrates the fact that individuals preferring the insertor role in fellatio tend to have become homosexually active earlier and to have been homosexually active longer than those without this pref-

TABLE 7.2 Psychosocial Variables Associated with Fellatio-insertor Role in Four-Country Sample

	No Preference	Prefer
Years education	12.4	11.1*
Time since became homosexually active	9.4	11.6+
Age homosexually active	20.7	19.1*
Homosexuality violates conventional morality[a]	3.4	4.0*
Homosexuality violates conformity in general[a]	3.1	3.6*
Self-rating:[a]		
Feminine	3.8	3.4+
Large penis	3.8	3.3+
Casual	4.6	4.2+
Preferred partner:[a]		
Intelligent	5.2	5.5+
Feminine	4.5	4.8+
Fat	4.3	3.9*
Casual	4.5	4.0+
Acceptance of own homosexuality	6.5	6.2**

[a]0-8 scale
+$p < .1$
*$p < .05$
**$p < .01$

erence. Suggestive of a view that those preferring the insertor role are less happy about their homosexuality are the indications that these individuals believe homosexuality to violate conventional morality and conformity in general more, and to accept their homosexuality less. Such individuals interestingly rate themselves as less feminine, and their preferred partners as more feminine, suggesting that tied in with the lack of acceptance of the homosexuality is a belief that is it "feminine" to take the insertee role. Interestingly, Riess (1961) noted that male hustlers were prepared to accept insertor roles in sexual interactions but refused to define themselves as homosexual or do anything that might be defined as "feminine," with homosexuality and femininity being equated. The characteristics of those who prefer the fellatio-insertor situation match Riess's findings in this regard.

Characteristics of those who prefer the fellatio-insertee practice provide an interesting contrast (Table 7.3). Again, lower formal education levels predict a preference for this practice, and the age respondents realized that they were homosexual and the age they became actively homosexual are both lower than the no-preference group. The aspect of sex role, however, mirror the previous group since insertees regard themselves as more passive and feminine, and rate as less masculine on the BSRI. Preferred partners tend to be less feminine, and the characteristic "involved," as was the case for the characteristic "casual" in the insertors, is reversed for partner suggesting the preference for complementarity in partners (as would be necessary for specific preferences to be matched). Again in mirror image, insertees see the laws and people in their country as being less antihomosexual, and are more likely to report that their relationships work on the basis of dominant-submissive roles. The influence of mother and teachers on behavior is less than those with no preference. Of particular interest is the fact that they are more likely to have seen a psychiatrist both about their homosexuality and about other matters. Taking these data together, the picture emerges that the individual who prefers the fellatio-insertee role is of individuals who see themselves as passive and feminine, and who appear to operate on the basis of mimicry of a heterosexual feminine role. Given that such a traditional role of involves devaluation of the self, it is not surprising that psychiatric help has been sought.

Characteristics of those who prefer fellatio but have no role preference are illustrated in Table 7.4. They are likely to be more homosexual in practice, to have had less negative reaction to their homosexuality, and to be more

TABLE 7.3 Psychosocial Variables Associated with Fellatio-insertee Role in Four-Country Sample

	% No Preference	% Prefer
Years education	12.5	10.1**
Influence of mother of behavior[a]	4.8	3.5**
Influence of teachers of behavior[a]	3.1	2.4*
Self-rating:[a]		
Passive	4.0	4.5+
Involved	3.9	3.4
Feminine	3.4	4.0*
Facial hair	3.8	4.4+
Preferred partner:[a]		
Extroverted	6.4	5.8+
Involved	4.0	3.6
Feminine	3.2	3.7+
Cold	2.6	2.3+
Masculinity	2.2	2.0+
Believes laws in own country antihomosexual compared with other places[a]	3.6	3.1*
Believes people in own country antihomosexual compared with other places[a]	3.9	3.2**
Time since became actively homosexual	9.5	11.7
Actual societal reaction against homosexuality	32.0	36.8*
Age became actively homosexual	20.7	19.0*
Age realized was homosexual	15.1	12.8
Relationships work on the basis of dominant-submissive roles	25.0	50.0
Seen psychiatrist about homosexuality	15.9	38.8**
Seen psychiatrist about anything else	21.9	34.0

[a]0-8 scale
+p < .1
*p < .05
**p < .01

masculine on the BSRI and more accepting of their homosexuality. They have significantly more partners (as might be expected given no role preference to influence partner selection), and see themselves as less passive and feminine. They have also been influenced by their fathers more, are less likely to have a religious commitment, less likely to have relationships working on the basis on any roles, and less likely to have seen a psychiatrist. The picture that

TABLE 7.4 Psychosocial Variables Associated with Both Fellatio Roles in Four-Country Sample

	% No Preference	% Prefer
Position on Kinsey Scale	5.2	5.4**
Actual societal reaction against homosexuality	35.4	31.4**
Believes people in own country antihomosexual compared to other places[a]	3.7	3.9
Number of partners per month average in past year	1.1	1.3**
Influence of father on behavior[a]	3.0	3.5*
Age realized people think homosexuality wrong	13.5	13.9
Self-rating:[a]		
Passive	4.3	3.0+
Feminine	3.7	3.4**
Short	4.3	4.1
Preferred partner:[a]		
Emotional	4.2	4.4+
Fat	4.0	3.7*
Acceptance of own homosexuality	6.3	6.6**
Masculinity	2.1	2.3**
Religious:		
Practicing	22.8	17.5
None	28.4	39.3
Relationships work on the basis of roles	22.1	14.2
Relationships work on basis of sexual roles only	40.0	14.7
Seen psychiatrist about homosexuality	24.5	15.1
Seen psychiatrist about anything else	28.1	20.9

[a]0-8 scale
+p < .1; *p < .05; **p < .01

emerges of those who prefer fellatio but have no preference as to insertor or insertee role is of more active and accepting individuals who, as expected, do not work on the basis of roles in relationships and who apparently have less problems that would require professional consultation.

In general, with fellatio it is clear that role preferences are coexisting with beliefs about many other roles, including sex roles and the homosexual role. Those who prefer fellatio regardless of role tend to be more accepting of their sexuality and less concerned about deviation from conventional male norms.

Anal Intercourse

Anal intercourse is associated in most people's minds with male homosexuality, and insertor and insertee preferences are often equated with male and female role playing. However, from Table 7.5 it is clear that less than 20 percent of homosexual men in this sample prefer one or the other, and less than 50 percent prefer both. It is thus less popular than fellatio and full body contact and, in Australia and Ireland, than mutual masturbation.

While the data (Table 7.5) on those respondents who prefer the anal intercourse-insertor role do confirm the linkage of this activity to sex roles, they also show that such individuals are older, have more partners and more STD infections than those with no preference, see themselves as typically masculine (not passive, more facial hair and shorter hair) and prefer partners who are the opposite (that is, typically more effeminate). They score as more masculine on the BSRI, realized that they were homosexual later than others (perhaps a function of not fitting the typically homosexual "feminine" stereotype), and do not believe that people in their country are particularly anti-homosexual, which suggests that their preference for an insertor role is not a reaction to stigmatism. Apart from these points, however, there is nothing to suggest that those preferring the anal-insertor role are dissimilar to those without such a role preference.

Similarly, the respondent with a preference for the insertee role in anal intercourse (Table 7.6) expect a less negative reaction to their homosexuality. They also expect a less negative societal reaction to their sexual orientation, but believe that the laws in their country are more anti-homosexual than other places. In direct contrast to those preferring the insertor role, they rate as less masculine on the BSRI and see themselves as more feminine, while pre-ferring, as expected, partners who are less passive. As with the individuals who had role preferences in fellatio, we find that outside the not unexpected sex role associations, there are no clear covarying factors that might explain these behavioral preferences. However, as with the fel-latio-insertee group, there is a marked preference for roles in relationships and the evidence that there has been more distress to the point where psychiatric consultation is necessary. Those preferring the anal-insertor role tend more often to be less well educated and to make more sexual contacts through their work, suggesting that their occupa-tion may also be one relating to traditional sex roles or stereotypes about homosexuality.

TABLE 7.5 Psychosocial Variables Associated with Anal Intercourse-insertor Role in Four-Country Sample

	% No Preference	% Prefer
Age	30.0	31.3
Numbers of partners per month--		
average in past year	1.2	1.4**
Times had STD infection	0.9	1.4*
Age realized people think homosexuality wrong	13.6	14.2+
Self-rating:[a]		
Passive	4.2	3.6**
Facial hair	3.5	4.2+
Short hair	6.1	5.4**
Delicate	5.6	5.2*
Preferred partner:[a]		
Sexy	4.8	4.6
Passive	3.6	4.6*
Extroverted	6.4	6.0*
Involved	4.1	3.8+
Feminine	3.2	3.5*
Smooth	5.0	5.5*
Facial hair	4.0	4.4+
Short hair	5.9	4.7**
Masculinity	2.2	2.4**
Believes people in own country antihomosexual		
compared to other places	3.6	3.3*
Ever engaged to be married	14.8	22.8*
Sexual contacts friends	32.3	41.4+

[a] 0-8 scale
+$p < .1$
*$p < .05$
**$p < .01$

Those respondents indicating that they preferred anal intercourse in both roles (Table 7.7) also differ from those with a role preference. They tend to be younger, to have been homosexually active for less time, and to have more partner per month on average than those with no preference. They also have had more STDs, and believe that homosexuality does not violate conformity in general to such a great extent, and are more accepting of their own homosexuality. This latter finding parallels the data on fellatio. On self-rating, those preferring both modes of anal inter-

TABLE 7.6 Psychosocial Variables Associated with Anal Intercourse-insertee Role in Four-Country Sample

	% No Preference	% Prefer
Years education	12.6	10.4**
Expected negative societal reaction against homosexuality	52.9	49.8*
Age became actively homosexual	20.8	19.0**
Self-rating:[a]		
Extroverted	5.7	5.2*
Feminine	3.4	4.0**
Short hair	6.0	5.4**
Preferred partner:[a]		
Passive	3.8	3.2**
Short	4.1	3.6**
Masculinity	2.5	2.0**
Believes laws in own country antihomosexual compared with other places[a]	4.4	4.9**
Relationships work on basis of male-female roles	10.5	29.2
Relationships work on basis of dominant-submissive roles	24.1	41.7+
Seen psychiatrist about homosexuality	16.0	28.8**
Sexual contact through work	4.0	9.1+

[a]0-8 scale
+p < .1
*p < .05
**p < .01

course describe themselves as more extroverted, less feminine, and more casual than those without such a preference, and as having more facial hair. Preferred partners are described as being casual, with less facial hair, and having similar interests. These data suggest that there is not such a polarity between self and partner as occurs in the individuals who prefer one mode of anal intercourse to the other. Of particular interest is the fact that those with a preference for both modes of anal intercourse score as higher on *both* masculinity and femininity on the BSRI (that is, are androgynous) than those with no preference. As might be expected from the data on fellatio that parallel these data, respondents who equally prefer insertor and insertee anal intercourse are less likely to have relationships that work on the basis of male-female or dominant-

TABLE 7.7 Psychosocial Variables Associated with Both Anal Intercourse Roles in Four-Country Sample

	% No Preference	% Prefer
Age	31.0	29.3**
Time since became homosexually active	10.3	9.0
Actual societal reaction against homosexuality	33.9	31.0*
Number of partner per month average in past year	1.2	1.3+
Times had STD infection	0.9	1.1+
Homosexuality violates conformity in general [a]	3.3	3.0*
Influence of female peers on behavior [a]	2.0	1.4*
Self-rating: [a]		
Extroverted	5.5	5.7+
Feminine	3.6	3.3*
Fat	3.9	3.6*
Facial hair	3.6	4.0*
Casual	4.4	4.7*
Preferred partner: [a]		
Facial hair	4.2	3.9*
Short hair	5.5	5.9*
Casual	4.2	4.6*
Similar interests	3.2	3.5*
Acceptance of own homosexuality	6.4	6.6*
Masculinity	2.2	2.3*
Femininity	2.8	2.9
Relationships work on basis of male-female roles	26.6	1.5**
Relationships work on basis of dominant-		
submissive roles	39.1	16.2**
Alternation of roles	64.8	81.6*

[a] 0-8 scale
+p < .1
*p < .05
**p < .01

submissive roles, and are more likely in fact to alternate the roles (or, more specifically, not to see them in terms of roles at all).

Comparison of the data on both fellatio and anal intercourse reveals some interesting findings. Little distinguishes the individuals with particular preferences from those with no preference apart from a strong preference for rigid roles and a dislike of nonstructured sexual behavior.

Such a preference for using tradition male-female roles, however, does have mental health implications, and as expected more of those in the "female" (submissive) role had seen a psychiatrist for problems relating to both their homosexuality and to other issues. Those who are happy to accept either insertor or insertee roles also tend to be more accepting of their homosexuality: this suggests that those who prefer only one role are less able to deal with stressors than androgynous individuals. In the case of the respondents who prefer the insertor role only in fellatio, there is also an indication that this role tends to allow them to deny that they are homosexual in the sense that they do not fit a stereotypical homosexual role. These data, taken together, however, do not suggest that sexual practices insofar as they are role related, have psychological determinants that are modifiable. However, the data do suggest that preferences for particular roles may be related to the degree of differentiation in the homosexual subculture and the length of time spent in that subculture. Those with role-related preferences tend to have been in the homosexual subculture longer than those with no role preference. This could imply that either role as related to sexual activities develop as a result of socialization, or that more probably the older homosexual men were socialized into the homosexual subculture at a time when roles were more common and when societal homosexual stereotypes were more prevalent.

Mutual Masturbation

The significance of a preference for mutual masturbation has vastly increased with the advent of AIDS, since this is a sexual practice in which there is no risk for transmission of pathogens unless ejaculation takes place in a body cavity (which would then classify as either fellatio or anal intercourse). Its significance as a means of reducing risk is evident by the rapid development in the United States of "Jack-off" locales which act as an outlet for safe alternatives to unsafe sexual practices.

There are some interesting contrasts (Table 7.8) between a preference for mutual masturbation and for the role-related sexual activities already described. Men who prefer mutual masturbation tend to be older, better educated, and became homosexually active later than those who do not prefer this activity. They tend to see people in their country as being more antihomosexual, and homosexuality as violating religious morality more. On the other hand, those preferring mutual masturbation also had a more positive societal reaction to their homosexuality from significant others. They were also likely to have been little influenced by male or female peers in contrast to those with no preference, which suggests that conventional socialization into sex roles had little effect on them compared with those who prefer the role-linked behaviors previously described in this chapter. Supporting this is the finding that such individuals spent less time in the homosexual subculture when they first became homosexually active, which may also have led to less socialization into a homosexual role.

It is particularly interesting to note in Table 7.8 that there are eight self-descriptors that differentiate those with a preference for mutual masturbation as a sexual practice, but only one preferred partner characteristic. Self-descriptions classify those with such a preference as less conventional, less passive, more intelligent and involved, and physically as having a smoother body, less facial hair and longer hair, and being more delicate. In contrast, the only characteristic preferred in a partner is the salient physical characteristic of penile size, but interestingly it is a preference for smaller than larger dimensions. As might also be expected, those preferring this sexual practice are less likely to have relationships working on the basis on any roles (particularly male-female roles) and to alternate any roles that do exist. Of particular interest is the fact that a greater proportion of those with a preference for mutual masturbation are likely to have monogamous relationships, another low risk for STD infection. However, there is surprisingly no significant difference in STD infection rate between groups.

These data are particularly interesting in that they suggest that those who do prefer mutual masturbation are better educated and are less socialized into both heterosexual sex roles and homosexual roles, possibly because of coexisting belief that homosexuality is more socially stigmatized. They also suggest that partner characteristics are less important for those individuals who prefer this practice, and that roles are also of no importance. Indeed, the picture that emerges strongly suggests that these individuals are not driven by particular partner needs or by particular internal models of social relationships: rather, this sexual behavior occurs often in monogamous relationships without an imposed structure. We can, with considerable confidence, use these data as an indication of some of the variables that might be emphasized to alter preferred behaviors from high risk to low risk of STD infection.

TABLE 7.8 Psychosocial Variables Associated with Mutual Masturbation in Four-Country Sample

	% No Preference	% Prefer
Age	29.7	30.6
Years education	11.8	12.7*
Actual societal reaction against homosexuality	33.9	31.2*
Age became homosexually active	20.1	20.9+
Believes people in own country antihomosexual compared with other places[a]	3.9	4.3**
Homosexuality violates religious (Christian) morality[a]	3.6	4.1**
Influence of male peers on behavior[a]	3.7	3.5*
Influence of female peers on behavior[a]	2.0	2.3*
Self-rating:[a]		
Conventional	4.8	4.6+
Passive	4.2	4.0
Intelligent	4.9	5.0+
Involved	3.7	4.0*
Smooth	5.0	5.2
Facial hair	4.0	3.7*
Short hair	6.1	5.7*
Delicate	5.4	5.6*
Preferred partner:[a]		
Large penis	4.2	4.0
% time spent in homosexual subculture when first became homosexually active	60.5	58.1
Relationships work on basis of any roles	21.1	12.3+
Relationships work on basis of male-female roles	28.8	16.9+
Alternation of roles	60.8	84.6**
Relationship monogamous	43.9	64.5**
Sexual contacts through work	2.8	6.5

[a]0-8 scale
+p < .1
*p < .05
**p < .01

Full Body Contact

Full body contact covers a variety of sexual behaviors, but most importantly refers to the degree of contact between individuals: it also implies a closer degree of emotional contact for the period of the sexual interaction at least, and a desire for sexual interaction rather than just sexual release. As a sexual practice, however, it describes the achieving of orgasm by mutual friction between two bodies. Reference to Table 7.9 reveals that individuals preferring full body contact tend to be older, realized they were homosexual later, and have become homosexually active later than those with no such preference. Of great interest is the fact that while those preferring full body contact tended to have more partners on average, they had significantly less STD infection. These data imply that full body contact may function as a form of sexual release more frequently than as an indicator of closeness of interaction, and that this sexual activity (a form of full-body masturbation) is of significantly lower risk than any other set of practices, including mutual masturbation. This may be because mutual masturbation takes place more frequently as a method of foreplay than as a method of achieving orgasm. While those preferring full body contact have had a more benign reaction to their homosexuality from significant others, they report a better relationship with their mother and that their father had a greater influence on their behavior than those without such a preference. This could suggest that their model of relationships could owe more to the parental model (which tends to emphasize physical proximity) than to models provided by peers or in the homosexual subculture. In common with those preferring mutual masturbation, there are major discrepancies in numbers of self-descriptors and of preferred partner characteristics, which also suggests that particular partner attributes are unimportant. Self-ratings for those preferring full body contact suggest than these individuals are more emotional, warm and extroverted, and see themselves as less passive but more delicate. They also, interestingly, prefer similarly less conventional partners, a finding that reinforces the suggestion that their models for sexual relationships are not conventionally homosexual or heterosexual, as does their lower score on sex role conservatism. The high score on femininity as measured by the BSRI, indicating a greater affective ability in interactions, also confirms that those preferring full body contact are interested in emotional as well as physical closeness in sexual interactions. Perhaps surprisingly, those preferring full body contact are less likely to have had a homosexual relationship lasting more than two years, and report that relationships are less likely to work on male-female roles and if roles occur, they are likely to be domestic only.

These data thus confirm that full body contact functions as an indicator of emotional as well as physical closeness,

TABLE 7.9 Psychosocial Variables Associated with Full Body Contact in Four-Country Sample

	% No Preference	% Prefer
Age	28.5	30.7**
Actual societal reaction against homosexuality	34.8	31.8*
Age became homosexually active	19.4	20.8**
Age realized was homosexual	14.0	15.1+
Number of partners per month average in past year	1.1	1.2
Times infected with STD	1.4	0.8*
Bad relationship with mother	3.4	3.0*
Influence of father on behavior	3.0	3.4*
Self-rating:[a]		
Emotional	4.1	4.5*
Conventional	5.0	4.6*
Passive	4.3	4.0
Extroverted	5.3	5.7*
Cold	3.3	2.8**
Large penis	3.4	3.8*
Delicate	5.2	5.6*
Preferred partner:[a]		
Conventional	5.0	4.6*
Femininity	2.7	2.9**
Sex role conservatism	34.3	36.2+
Had homosexual relationship more than 2 years	53.9	42.2*
Relationships based on domestic roles only	33.6	23.7*
Relationships work on basis of male-female roles	3.1	17.5+

[a] 0-8 scale
+p < .1
*p < .05
**p < .01

and that if used as a means of achieving orgasm is associated with a lower risk of STD infection. The lack of association with conventional roles also suggests that individuals who prefer this mode of sexual activity have not been socialized into the patterns of their peers during adolescence nor into homosexual roles that mimic heterosexuals. Rather they appear to see sexual relationships in terms of emotional and physical proximity, although there is no indication that such relationships last longer than those with no such preference. The lower rate of STD infection, however, confirms that this sexual practice is at a significantly lower risk than the other sexual activities described in this chapter.

Sadomasochistic Practices

Sadomasochistic practices have recently received more attention, with a greater recognition of both their occurrence and the dangers associated with them. In the present four-country sample, preference for sadomasochistic practices constituted abound 10 percent of all cases, which is a significant proportion of the total, and are not significantly biased toward any of the cultures in this sample. Risks from sadomasochistic practices in terms of STD infection are twofold. Where brachioproctic eroticism ("fist-fucking") is practiced, there is a significantly increased risk of rectal tears that may act as a portal for entry of pathogens if anal intercourse follows. Lesions further up the gastrointestinal tract carry a major risk of hemorrhage or peritonitis, especially given the paucity of sentient nerve fibers in the innervation of the colon. As a consequence, any lesions are likely to go undetected, especially if the use of drugs to assist in brachioproctic dilation has occurred. If other sadomasochistic practices lead to contact between body fluids such as blood, semen, saliva or urine, and mucous membranes, then there is also a risk of infection with a variety of pathogens. There is, however, not an great deal of literature on sexually transmitted pathogens and sadomasochistic practices.

Table 7.10 lists the variables that significantly discriminated between those with a preference for sadomasochistic practices and those with no such preference. Those who prefer sadomasochistic practices were younger when they realized they were homosexual, became homosexually active at a younger age, and had been homosexually active longer than those without such a preference. They also had more partners per month on average and a very significantly higher number of STD infections: interestingly, they saw homosexuality as violating religious morality *less* but conformity in general *more* than the comparison group. Perhaps this result comes about because of the view that their preferred sexual practice also appears to violate some of the norms of the homosexual subculture, which still has very ambivalent attitudes to sadomasochism, but sadomasochistic practices are not referred to in religious texts.

Supporting this is the self-rating of those preferring sadomasochistic practices as less conventional. Other self-ratings suggest that they also see themselves as being more sexy, more intelligent, more involved, colder, with shorter hair, and less passive than the comparison group. Preferred partners were also seen as being less conventional, heavier and with shorter hair, suggesting a recognition of people with shared interests by appearance or apparent unconventionality. As might be expected from the popular stereotype, those with sadomasochistic preferences were more masculine on the BSRI, and less sex role conservative. Interestingly, more were practicing in a religion, which may also explain their views of homosexuality as being less violating of religious morality. Consistent also with the view of sadomasochistic practices as involving role-taking, all indicated that their relationships were based on dominant-submissive roles, and more made sexual contacts through friends or cruising. Given that sadomasochistic sexual practices have until recently attracted much of the approbrium that was directed toward homosexuality several decades ago, it is not unexpected that those preferring sadomasochistic practices were more likely than those without such a preference to have seen a psychiatrist either about their sexuality or about other matters.

Sadomasochistic sexual activities appear to have a high risk of STD infection and are associated particularly with unconventional (to many homosexuals and heterosexuals) dominant-submissive roles and higher partner numbers. Such individuals as prefer this activity found they became homosexually aware and homosexually involved at a much younger age than those without such a preference, and are more masculine and less sex role conservative than their comparison group. It would appear that sadomasochistic sexual practices are related to a role preference not for conventional male-female roles but to a different type of role in which dominance and submission are integral needs. There are, however, no indications that particular psychological characteristics are associated with this sexual practice, contrary to popular belief.

SOUTH AUSTRALIAN SAMPLE

A number of hypotheses might be raised from the data presented so far. These include whether parental models have any influence on sexual practices, and precisely what STDs are associated with particular behaviors. Are particular mood states indicators of sexual activity? Can the findings of the associations of particular sexual practices with social, demographic, and psychological variables be replicated in a new sample? These are all questions that

TABLE 7.10 Psychosocial Variables Associated with Sadomasochistic Practices in Four-Country Sample

	% No Preference	% Prefer
Time since became homosexually active	9.3	12.2*
Age became homosexually active	20.7	19.3
Age realized was homosexual	15.1	13.1*
Number of partners per month average in past year	1.2	1.4+
Times infected with STD	0.9	1.9**
Homosexuality violates religious (Christian) morality	3.9	3.4+
Homosexuality violates conformity in general	4.8	5.2+
Self-rating:[a]		
Conventional	4.8	4.2*
Sexy	3.7	4.3**
Passive	4.1	3.7*
Intelligent	4.9	5.2
Involved	3.8	4.4*
Cold	2.7	3.0*
Short hair	5.2	6.0**
Preferred partner:[a]		
Conventional	4.8	4.2*
Fat	3.7	4.0+
Short hair	4.9	5.8**
Masculinity	2.2	2.3*
Sex role conservatism	3.6	3.4
Religious:		
Practicing	17.4	31.3
Nominal	46.5	31.3
Relationships work on basis of dominant-submissive roles	67.6	100.0
Seen psychiatrist about homosexuality	16.8	25.8
Seen psychiatrist about anything else	21.7	32.8*
Sexual contacts through cruising	15.6	21.1**
Sexual contacts through friends	32.2	47.1**

[a] 0-8 scale
+$p < .1$
*$p < .05$
**$p < .01$

may be answered by a briefer look at the associations of sexual practices in the South Australian sample, and additionally provide a deeper perspective on the determinants of particular sexual activities.

Fellatio (Direction Unspecified)

Table 7.11 lists the variables that distinguish between those who scored above and below the median (5) on an eight-point scale on which respondents scored their frequency of fellatio in sexual encounters. The table shows some interesting distinctions between low- and high-frequency fellators, particularly on parental rearing patterns: first, that the most negative parental rearing patterns are associated with low frequency of fellation in sexual encounters. Second, six of the nine patterns relate to the mother. These data strongly suggest that for fellatio, more rejecting, depriving and abusive parents who favor the siblings over the respondent depress sexual activity, possibly through damage to the individual's self-concept. The fact that the mother is more strongly implicated in fellatio does lend some support to the psychoanalytic belief that mothers are associated with oral gratification, and that an abusive and punitive mother may damage or suppress the expression of oral gratification in individuals. In this regard it is interesting that mood states as measured on the POMS confirm that low-frequency fellators are more angry and hostile, confused, tense and fatigued than those reporting a high frequency. This may be a direct result of negative parenting patterns, and also confirms that fellatio is associated with hedonistic rather than depressed psychological state.

Those respondents with high fellatio frequency also report higher partner numbers on average and spend more time in the homosexual subculture, and tend to meet partners in saunas (bath houses) more frequently. They also use marijuana more frequently. STD incidence reveals that high-frequency fellators are more likely to have had anal and penile gonorrhea, anal warts, nongonococcal urethritis (NSU), and herpes of the lips, but less likely to have had herpes zoster (shingles). Since only three of these STDs are possibly related to fellatio, it must be concluded that high-frequency fellators are also likely to have a high frequency of other sexual activities. As might be expected, the high-frequency fellators have a very significantly increased rate of STD infection over the past one and five years.

These data do suggest that parental, especially maternal, rearing patterns have an influence on fellation, and

TABLE 7.11 Psychosocial Variables Associated with Sexual Practices in South Australian Sample

	Low Frequency	High Frequency
Fellatio (direction unspecified)		
Parental rearing pattern:		
Father abusive	10.4	8.7*
Mother abusive	9.8	8.3*
Father depriving	11.9	9.8**
Mother depriving	11.2	9.6**
Mother punitive	14.5	12.6
Mother rejecting	14.8	13.2*
Mother overinvolved	16.6	15.0+
Father favors siblings	8.4	7.0+
Mother favors siblings	8.1	6.6*
Mood states:		
Anger-Hostility	23.2	19.8*
Confusion	15.4	13.5*
Tension	21.6	18.2*
Fatigue	18.2	14.7**
Partners per month past year	2.6	4.7*
% time spent in homosexual subculture	34.7	44.7*
Rank position: meet partners at work	2.6	4.0*
Rank position: meet partners at sauna	2.6	2.0*
Marijuana: times past year	1.0	2.9**
Marijuana: times past 5 years	1.1	3.3*
Penile gonorrhea past 5 years	0.0	0.1*
Anal gonorrhea past year	0.0	0.1*
Herpes lips past year	0.0	0.1+
Shingles past year	0.1	0.0*
Anal warts past year	0.0	0.1+
NSU past year	0.0	0.2*
Times had STD infection past year	0.2	0.7**
Times had STD infection past 5 years	1.3	2.5**
Anal Intercourse-Insertor		
Parental rearing pattern:		
Mother punitive	13.8	12.6+
Father affectionate	11.7	10.7*
Father performance-oriented	12.7	11.7+
Father stimulating	11.5	10.1*
Masculinity	1.0	1.3*
Femininity	1.7	1.4*
Mood state: fatigue	17.3	14.0**
Self-esteem	37.0	39.3*
Homosexual self-esteem	37.2	39.1*
Age	31.7	34.7*

123

TABLE 7.11   Continued

	Low Frequency	High Frequency
% time spent in homosexual subculture	37.5	46.5*
Years homosexually active	11.3	14.3*
Drinks alcohol per day past 5 years	2.9	2.1*
Volatile nitrites past 5 years	1.3	2.4*
Depressed past 3 months[a]	3.2	2.3**
Penile gonorrhea past year	0.0	0.1+
Penile gonorrhea past 5 years	0.1	0.2*
Hepatitis past year	0.1	0.0
Herpes penis past year	0.1	0.0*
Times STD infection past 5 years	1.6	2.6*
Anal Intercourse-Insertee		
Parental rearing pattern:		
Father abusive	8.7	9.8+
Father rejecting	15.2	16.9*
% time spent in homosexual subculture	37.0	47.0*
Rank position: meet partners at bars	2.3	1.8*
Rank position: meet partners cruising	1.8	2.4*
Rank position: meet partners at work	3.9	3.0*
Rank position: meet partners through friends	2.3	1.9*
Oral gonorrhea past 5 years	0.0	0.1*
Anal gonorrhea past year	0.1	0.2*
Shingles past year	0.1	0.0*
Mutual Mastuerbation		
Parental rearing pattern:		
Father abusive	10.0	8.0**
Father depriving	10.9	9.5**
Mother depriving	10.4	9.6*
Father punitive	14.8	12.1**
Father shaming	8.4	6.9**
Father rejecting	17.3	14.0**
Mother rejecting	14.7	12.1**
Father tolerant	16.7	19.0**
Mother tolerant	17.2	19.3**
Father affectionate	10.6	12.1**
Father guilt-engendering	8.7	7.7*
Father stimulating	9.9	12.2**
Mother stimulating	11.5	13.3**
Father favors siblings	8.3	6.2**
Years homosexually active	13.8	11.3+
Penile gonorrhea past year	0.1	0.0*
Shingles past year	0.1	0.0*
Times had STD infection past year	0.6	0.3*
Times had STD infection past 5 years	2.5	1.4*

TABLE 7.11 Continued

	Low Frequency	High Frequency
Analingus-Insertor		
Parental rearing pattern:		
Mother rejecting	14.5	13.0+
Mother tolerant	17.6	18.7*
Mother affectionate	11.8	12.8*
Mother stimulating	11.5	12.9*
Mother favors respondent	6.8	7.9*
Mood states:		
Anger-hostility	22.3	19.5*
Friendliness	21.0	22.9*
Tension	20.4	18.0+
Fatigue	16.8	14.7+
Homosexual self-esteem	36.8	39.3**
Time spent in homosexual subculture	37.2	45.2+
Rank position: meet partners at work	2.8	4.1**
Alcohol drinks per day past year	2.1	2.9*
Oral gonorrhea past 5 years	0.0	0.1*
Hepatitis past year	0.0	0.1*
Herpes lips past year	0.2	0.1*
Penile herpes past year	0.0	0.1*
Shingles past year	0.1	0.0*
Times STD infection past year	0.3	0.7*
Times STD infection past 5 years	1.6	2.5*

[a] 0-8 scale
+p < .1
*p < .05
**p < .01

that negative mood state also has a strong relationship with this particular sexual activity. More frequent fellation is linked to higher incidence of STD infection.

Anal Intercourse-Insertor

Reference to Table 7.11 reveals that parental rearing patterns also play a part in frequency of insertor anal intercourse, but that in this case it is the father's pattern that is the better predictor. Fathers who are more affectionate, performance-oriented, and stimulating are associated with a *lower* frequency of anal insertor sex. This tends to suggest that a high frequency of this sexual practice (median = 4) is linked to a negative paternal rearing pattern, and in a psychodynamic formulation this could suggest that anal intercourse in the insertor role, at least in high frequencies, is a masculine overcompensation for lack of paternal warmth. This is supported by the fact that high masculinity and low femininity as measured on the BSRI are also associated with high frequency of this particular sexual activity. A more parsimonious explanation, however, would be suggested by social learning theory, since the traditional male parent is not expected to display a positive affect, and this may explain the hypermasculinity in the son.

As found in the four-country study, those with a preference for insertor anal intercourse tend to be older and spend more time in the homosexual subculture. In common with the findings on fellatio, negative mood states such as fatigue and depression are linked with a low sexual frequency. Drug use suggests that anal insertors use less alcohol but more volatile nitrites, and STD infection rates suggest that they are at greater risk for penile gonorrhea, but lower risk for hepatitis and penile herpes. However, they do have an increased STD infection rate over those with low anal insertor frequency. These data again implicate psychodynamic factors in that those with a high frequency of this practice have higher self-esteem and self-esteem as homosexuals, but whether this is cause or effect of a high frequency of anal insertor sex is not possible to determine.

Anal Intercourse-Insertee

Few psychosocial variables were associated with a high frequency of anal-insertee sex (median = 2). The only parental rearing patterns implicated are, as in anal insertor sex, linked to a negative father. Again, psychodynamically this could be interpreted as an attempt to replace the father by another male, but the pattern is weak and should not be overemphasized. Anal insertee preference is associated with a higher proportion of time spent in the homosexual subculture, and with meeting partners in bars and at work more frequently, and cruising less frequently.

Surprisingly, there were few STD infections associated with a higher frequency of insertee anal intercourse in this sample, with a higher reported rate of oral and anal gonorrhea, and a lower frequency of shingles. These data appear contradictory when compared with the literature, which suggests that anal insertee intercourse is the most risk associated for STD infection. Clearly, this need not always be the case. However, the paucity of psychosocial correlates for this sexual practice does imply that it is not psychosocially determined to the degree it was anticipated, at least in this sample.

Mutual Masturbation

The STD consequences of a preference for mutual masturbation (median = 4) are quite clear from data in Table 7.11: those preferring this activity are at significantly lower risk than those without such a preference. Of particular interest, however, are the large number of parental rearing variables that are associated with this sexual behavior pattern. Again, it is apparently the father who is of greatest importance, with more than two-thirds of the significant variables referring to the father. In addition, most are highly significantly different between the high- and low-frequency groups. In all cases, the low frequency for mutual masturbation group had more punitive, shaming, rejecting, intolerant, and unaffectionate fathers, with the maternal variables showing the same trend. These data strongly suggest that there is a psychodynamic association between parental rearing patterns and a preference for mutual masturbation. The most likely explanation is that positive rearing by parents, particularly the father, may both endow the male genitals with a positive set of associations, make closer mutual interaction possible, and permit non-role-related sexual activities. These data may have considerable importance in attempting to modify sexual behaviors toward less risky alternatives, and do suggest that exploration of the meanings of sexual behavior may be of considerable use in some situations. These data also imply that role-related activities are associated with a greater time of being homosexually active, and that socialization into particular role preferences may occur.

Analingus-Insertor

One sexual activity that has not been examined in the four-country sample, but which has been implicated in transmission of enteric pathogens, is analingus. Reference to Table 7.11 shows a quite remarkable similarity in two ways to the data on fellatio. In both cases, maternal rearing patterns are implicated, and in both, mood states are also implicated. In the case of those preferring analingus (median = 1), maternal rearing variables follow an identical pattern to fellatio, with those with the most positive maternal patterns having a higher preference. It cannot be a coincidence that both oral sexual activities both show the same maternal rearing pattern, and the same association of mood states (with the more positive being associated with higher frequency of active analingus). It could probably be concluded that oral sexual activities are possible where mother-son interaction has permitted oral dependency needs to be met, thus imbuing oral activity with a positive set of connotations. In addition to this, negative mood states appear to mitigate against oral sexual activities, which suggests that these activities are hedonistically determined rather than meeting particular sexual needs. This is supported by the fact that those preferring analingus have higher homosexual self-esteem.

Those preferring analingus tend to have more alcoholic drinks per day, and to be less likely to meet sexual partners at work. The consequences of analingus for STD infection, however, are fairly consistent. They are more likely to have had hepatitis, herpes of the lips, and oral gonorrhea, as well as penile herpes: however, they are less likely to have had shingles. Over both one and five years, they are more likely to have had more STD infections than those without a preference for active analingus. These data do suggest that there may be more similarities than differences between analingus and fellatio, and that these similarities are based both on maternal rearing patterns and on mood states.

Insofar as these South Australian data deal with psychological variables such as parental rearing patterns and mood states, they provide a fascinating amplification of some of the determinants of particular sexual practices, and add to the understanding of why particular sexual practices are selected or rejected. Of course, probably the major determinant of sexual practices is partner, yet we can see from the four-country sample data that even partner characteristics may be selected to increase the probability of a particular sexual activity. These findings, in the case of some sexual activities at least, may aid the modification of at-risk behaviors to reduce the *probability* of STD infection.

In conclusion, it is apparent that there are a number of major psychological and social concommitants of particular sexual activities. Oral activities, including both fellatio and analingus, appear to be associated with maternal rearing patterns and mood states, suggesting that they may be related both to gratification of oral dependency needs and to hedonism. Insertor and insertee roles in both fellatio and anal intercourse appear to be strongly related to conventional masculine and feminine sex roles, and activities such as full-body contact and mutual masturbation are non-role related. It would appear that these last two activities occur when there is emphasis on emotional as well as physical closeness, and that they lead as expected to decreased frequencies of STD infection. The data also suggest that sexual socialization into homosexual subcultures and, to a lesser extent, parental and peer models, have a major influence on the type of sexual activities indulged in: increased socialization increases role specificity, as does degree of differentiation of the homosexual subculture within which that socialization occurs.

While modification of particular sexual activities may not be easy, there is some evidence that understanding the psychosocial bases of such activities may assist in attempting change.

8

Partner Anonymity and Places of Sexual Contact: Some Psychosocial Relationships

Partner anonymity and place of sexual contact play an important part in STD infection. While there is almost no literature available on these subjects, the links between STD infection and anonymity are twofold. First, the possibility of contact tracing is near to impossible given that partners may not be known, nor even recognized if contact took place in a darkened atmosphere. Second, in some places of anonymous contact there is an opportunity for multiple sexual acts with multiple partners, which increases the risk of infection in an exponential fashion if sexual partners have also had multiple partners. As an example, if an individual has four partners, and each of his partners has also had four partners, the risk of infection is increased at least 16-fold (more if each of the partner contacts have also had multiple sexual contacts). While in practice it is unlikely that this will occur, it is clear that risk of infection may be substantially increased. A third issue of more than passing interest is the link between high partner numbers and particular venues for anonymous sexual contacts such as saunas (referred to as bath houses in North America), back-room bars, and some cruising areas that encompass sheltering vegetation or public conveniences. Such places cater to those who wish for quick, anonymous sexual gratification, but it is not clear whether those seeking such gratification are using it as a means of avoiding close emotional contact with others, whether it is used for sexual release additional to close emotional contacts, or whether in many cases it is used by those who do not identify primarily as homosexual. Humphreys (1970)

last point in his major study of those seeking
ct in public conveniences, and found that some
of those making contact were married and for
art identified themselves as primarily hetero-

ys's study classified those using public conven-
laces for sexual gratification into four groups:
nbisexuals, gays, and closet queens. The
ip comprised married men who worked as truck
chine operators or clerical workers, and in 63
the marriages, both husband and wife were
olics. In this group, two-thirds took an in-
in fellatio in sexual encounters. Ambisexuals
d men with double the median income of the
ip, and usually Protestants. Two-thirds of this
insertees in fellatio. Such individuals saw
as bisexual, but were able to compartmentalize
orientations into heterosexual and homosexual
without much interaction or conflict between the two. The
gay group were individuals who were unmarried and had no
preference for sexual roles and who had independent occupations, while the "closet queens" are also unmarried but in
lower middle class occupations in which they were dependent on others for employment. They avoid homosexual
contacts in other places in the homosexual subculture, of
which they are not a part. Humphreys found that most of
these individuals preferred to play the insertor role, at
least until they lost their attractiveness, and half of this
group were Roman Catholics. While the "closet queens"
would appear to embody those individuals who avoid emotional contact, they clearly have little or no contact with
the homosexual subculture and thus do not appear in samples. This biases our data on those who make contacts
cruising to include only the "gay" group of Humphreys's
typology, and results must thus be treated with caution.
    Bell and Weinberg (1978) reported extensively on places
of cruising for sexual contact in homosexual men, and found
that 43 percent of their white respondents cruised once a
week or more frequently. Of those who sought sexual
partners, 66 percent went to bars, 54 percent to bath
houses, 48 percent on the street, 44 percent at private
parties, 30 percent in parks, 30 percent on beaches, 22
percent in public conveniences and 15 percent in movie
theatres. Frequency of seeking sexual contacts in each of
these locales was bars, 53 percent more than once a week;
bath houses, 15 percent more than once a week; streets, 39
percent more than once a week; private partners, 6 percent
more than once a week; parks, 27 percent more than once a

week; beaches, 21 percent more than once a week; public conveniences, 35 percent more than once a week; and movie theatres, 17 percent more than once a week. In terms of locations in which one-third or more of cruising time was spent, bars were the most common place (33 percent), followed by bath houses and the street (14 percent each). However, there is no indication of the degree of overlap in places of sexual partner contact, and as Bell and Weinberg point out, their data were gathered in the San Francisco Bay Area and their findings may not be representative of other areas which are not major cities with a reputation of being gay meccas.

What is perhaps of greatest importance in examining places of sexual contact from a psychovenereological standpoint is to make an assessment of the variables, both social and psychological, which are associated with choice of particular locales. While in the past this was of some interest from an academic standpoint in the understanding and classification of homosexual behavior, it has recently become clinically important. With the spread of AIDS within homosexual communities in the past few years, such information may serve to explain the forces that lead to homosexual men who prefer anonymous sexual encounters. If an understanding of the mechanisms that may underly choice of anonymous contacts can be reached, it may be possible to modify such behaviors to enable sexual contacts to carry less risk and to make contact tracing easier.

As with previous chapters, we will first examine the cultural determinants of preference for particular locales, and then examine the four-country sample in an attempt to discover cross-cultural variables that are associated with preference for particular locales. These have for convenience been divided into the less anonymous locales (bars and clubs, friends) and the more anonymous (beats, cruising). Work locale is added for comparison, but saunas (bath houses) are omitted from the four-country list since in Finland, saunas have nonsexual connotations, and there was no gay sauna in Ireland at the time of data collection. Stockholm had a semi-gay sauna, and there were also homosexual saunas in Melbourne and Brisbane. In the South Australian sample, however, the presence of a gay sauna made it possible to include this as a response category.

FOUR-COUNTRY SAMPLE

While it was anticipated that there would be few differences between the four countries in terms of place of sexual contacts, on all four variables (cruising, bars and clubs, work, and through friends), all but through friends showed significant differences. For cruising, the proportion decreased from Swedes at the highest percentage (Table 8.1) through to the Irish at the lowest percentage. This difference across countries tends to follow the degree of differentiation of the homosexual community from Sweden and Australia, where it is most differentiated, through to Finland and Ireland, where it is least differentiated. A similar pattern follows for making sexual contacts at work,

TABLE 8.1 Places of Sexual Contact in Four Countries

	No (%)	Yes (%)
Beats, Cruising		
Swedes	77.3	22.7
Australians	78.5	21.5
Finns	89.8	10.2
Irish	90.2	9.8**
Work		
Swedes	91.5	8.5
Australians	96.8	3.2
Finns	96.6	3.4
Irish	97.5	2.5*
Bars, Clubs		
Swedes	31.8	68.2
Australians	55.1	44.9
Finns	49.0	51.0
Irish	40.2	59.8**
Friends		
Swedes	63.1	36.9
Australians	63.3	36.7
Finns	66.0	34.0
Irish	73.8	26.2

*χ^2_4, $p < .05$
**χ^2_4, $p < .01$

which also suggests that the degree of differentiation of the gay scene might be the relevant determinant, since the ability to make contacts at place of work implies that place of work is a specifically homosexually oriented locale such as a bar, sauna, or gay business. On the other hand, it may also include occupations in which a high proportion of homosexual men are believed to work, such as waiting, but this is unlikely. The exception to the trend of higher contacts in the more homosexually differentiated countries is bars and clubs. In this case, the most contacts in bars and clubs are made by Swedes, followed in order of magnitude by Irish, Finns, and Australians. It is hard to explain these data, although it may be that there are more obviously homosexual bars and clubs in Stockholm and Dublin than in Helsinki, Melbourne, and Brisbane, but it would appear that this is not the case. However, in the other two sexual contact places, the data do suggest that the degree of development of the homosexual community may be an indicator of the frequency with which various locales are used for sexual contact.

The variables that differentiate those who do not make contact with partners while cruising known "beats" and those who do are illustrated in Table 8.2. Such individuals appear to have both mothers and teachers who had little influence on their behavior, but their male peers had more influence on such individuals, whereas peer pressure and the mores of the homosexual community may have more of an influence on the behavior of such individuals. Those who cruise "beats" (which include parks, streets, beaches, and public conveniences) describe themselves as more introverted, more well-built, more casual, and more rugged than those who do not cruise. In terms of genital attributes, they describe themselves as having smaller penises than noncruisers: it is interesting that they also prefer partners with smaller genitals, and particularly that preferred partner characteristics are for individuals who are more masculine and less delicate than noncruisers. These data suggest that those who cruise see themselves as being fairly well-built and rugged, and that they prefer masculine partners. Of some interest is the fact that cruisers describe themselves as introverted, suggesting that they may find emotional interaction too demanding. Those who cruise are more sex role conservative, which suggests that their belief in roles within homosexual relationships may be stronger, and have, as expected, significantly higher numbers of partners. They are, as also expected, less likely to be in a homosexual relationship at present that had lasted over two years, and that relationship is likely to be nonmonogamous if they are in one. Of interest is the fact that of those who have seen a psychiatrist for any reasons, cruisers are overrepresented: this may be related to views

TABLE 8.2 Psychosocial Variables Differentiating Individuals in Four
Countries Meeting Sexual Partners Cruising

	No Cruising	Cruising
Influence of mother on behavior[a]	4.3	3.6**
Influence of male peers on behavior[a]	3.5	4.0*
Influence of teachers and school on behavior[a]	3.2	2.7+
Self-rating:[a]		
Extroverted	5.7	5.1**
Fat	3.7	4.1*
Small penis	4.4	4.0*
Casual	4.5	5.0**
Delicate	5.6	5.0**
Preferred partner:[a]		
Feminine	3.3	2.8**
Small penis	4.0	3.3**
Delicate	5.3	4.3**
Sex role conservatism	35.1	39.4**
Partners per month average in past year	2.0	4.8**
% in homosexual relationship now 2 years:		
No	72.6	27.4
Yes	82.2	17.8*
% relationship is monogamous:		
No	56.4	43.6
Yes	39.3	60.7+
% ever seen psychiatrist for any reason:		
No	78.7	21.3
Yes	68.8	31.2*

[a]8-point scale
+$p < .075$
*$p < .05$
**$p < .01$

of sexuality or problems in relating to others, but there is
no clear evidence to implicate one or the other of these
speculations.

Table 8.3 gives those variables that distinguish those
who do from those who do not meet sexual partners at
work: it must be recalled, however, that the numbers of
those who meet sexual partners through work are small,
less than 5 percent of the total cases. Those individuals
who meet partners at work describe themselves as more
intelligent and warmer, and less passive and feminine. It

TABLE 8.3 Psychosocial Variables Differentiating Individuals in Four Countries Meeting Sexual Partners at Work

	Not at Work	At Work
Self-rating:[a]		
Passive	4.0	3.4**
Intelligent	4.9	5.3*
Feminine	3.5	3.0*
Cold	2.9	2.6+
Preferred partner:[a]		
Facial hair	4.1	2.9**
Casual	4.1	3.8+

[a] 8-point scale
+p < .075
*p < .05
**p < .01

would appear that such individuals believe that they fit conventional masculine norms to a greater degree, which suggests strongly that they are not part of the gay-stereotyped occupation group as previously postulated. Their preferred partners are more likely to be clean-shaven and casual, but this offers no clue as to their occupations. No further information distinguishes this group from those who do not make contact with sexual partners at work, so it must be assumed that they do not form a significantly different subgroup.

Psychosocial variables differentiating those who make sexual contacts in bars and clubs appear in Table 8.4. Individuals making sexual contacts in such places believe that homosexuality violates conformity in general less than do those who do not meet partners in bars and clubs, and this tends to confirm that those who do not use public, social locales are less accepting of their sexual orientation and believe it to be more nonconforming to social mores as a lifestyle. Similarly, those who use bars and clubs report that male peers are a greater influence on their behavior, which also suggests that bar-goers are more socialized into the public homosexual scene. On self-rating, bar and club attenders describe themselves as more emotional, sexy and passive, and less feminine, cold, well-built, and hairy. These data also confirm that bar and club goers have a greater interest in, or ability to, act in a warmer, more

TABLE 8.4 Psychosocial Variables Differentiating Individuals in Four
Countries Meeting Sexual Partners in Bars and Clubs

	Not in Clubs, Bars	Clubs, Bars
Homosexuality violates conformity in general[a]	3.3	3.0*
Influence of male peers on behavior[a]	3.4	3.7*
Self-rating:[a]		
Emotional	4.2	4.5*
Sexy	3.6	3.9*
Passive	4.2	3.9*
Feminine	3.6	3.3*
Cold	3.1	2.8*
Fat	4.0	3.6**
Smooth	5.3	5.0*
Preferred partner:[a]		
Intelligent	5.1	5.3+
Similar interests	3.2	3.5*
Extent laws in country prohomosexual,		
compared with other places[a]	4.3	4.5+
% leisure time spent in homosexual subculture	58.1	61.9**
% ever had homosexual relationship for		
more than 2 years:		
No	48.8	51.2
Yes	60.2	39.8**
% in homosexual relationship now more		
than 2 years:		
No	67.3	32.7
Yes	79.4	20.6**
% relationship is monogamous:		
No	39.1	60.9
Yes	55.6	44.4*

[a] 8-point scale
+$p < .075$
*$p < .05$
**$p < .01$

emotional fashion and that for this reason they prefer bars
and clubs in which there is a greater degree of social
contact and expressed affect. Preferred partner ratings
confirm this, with preferred partners being described as
those with greater intelligence and more similar interests:

both are factors that may only be assessed with some degree of social interaction. It would appear that, from these data, bar and club attenders do so because of a need for homosocial rather than just homosexual interaction. They are less likely to see homosexuality as being in violation of the laws of the country, and spend, as might be expected given their preference for social interaction with prospective partners, significantly more time in the homosexual subculture. In terms of relationship status, they are less likely to have been in a homosexual relationship for more than two years, and similarly less likely at the time of responding to be in a homosexual relationship that had been going for longer than two years. If they were in a homosexual relationship, it was more likely to be a nonmonogamous one.

These data confirm the popular expectation that homosexual men who seek sexual contacts in bars and clubs are more thoroughly socialized into the homosexual subculture, and see homosexuality as less a threat to society and less threatened by the laws in their country. This latter point suggests that those who congregate in the more public places such as known gay bars and clubs see their homosexual orientation as less negative than those who meet partners in other places. In particular, those who meet potential partners in bars and clubs appear to prefer to have a social and emotional level of interaction with their potential partners that is significantly greater than those who seek contacts in other places. To the homosexual man who frequents bars and clubs for sexual contact, then, the social and affective interaction is as important as the sexual one, and his preferred partner characteristics include interactional rather than physical attributes. This group, then, appear to make contacts with people with whom they interact at a social and emotional level and for this to probably be a necessary, although not sufficient, condition for a sexual liaison. It also suggests that there is a far greater potential for relationships to develop than in any of the other places of meeting sexual partners.

One would also expect individuals who met sexual partners through friends to follow this pattern, perhaps to an even greater degree. Table 8.5 illustrates those variables that significantly differentiated homosexual men who made sexual contacts through friends from those who did not. Those seeking partners among friends report that they realized that homosexuality was considered by others to be wrong significantly later than those not seeking partners among friends, and this does suggest that the negative view of many individuals in Western society about

TABLE 8.5 Psychosocial Variables Differentiating Individuals in Four
Countries Meeting Sexual Partners through Friends

	Not Through Friends	Through Friends
Age realized people think homosexuality wrong	13.5	14.2*
Self-rating:[a]		
Conventional	4.8	4.5*
Intelligent	5.1	5.3+
Socially involved	3.9	4.2+
Short hair	5.8	5.5*
Preferred partner:[a]		
Conventional	4.8	4.4**
Extroverted	5.5	5.8*
Socially involved	3.8	4.2**
Masculinity	2.2	2.3**
% leisure time spent in homosexual subculture	59.4	62.0+
Partners per month average past year	2.7	2.1**
% ever had homosexual relationship		
for more than 2 years:		
No	57.9	42.1
Yes	50.2	49.8+
% in homosexual relationship now more		
than 2 years:		
No	69.0	31.0
Yes	76.8	23.2*

[a] 8-point scale
+p < .075
*p < .05
**p < .01

homosexuality has not been internalized as early or as
strongly as in those who do not seek partners through
friendship networks. One could further speculate that for
this reason, sexual partners are seen as friends and com-
panions, and that this view of sexual contacts is closer to
the heterosexual model. It is possible that those who do
not meet partners through friends have internalized the
negative social attitudes toward homosexuality to the extent
where they can receive their sexual gratification this way,
but are unable to accept or maintain social gratification
homosexually. However, this may not be demonstrated in
the present study, and is a speculation which moves beyond

the scope of these data.

These data also confirm that social interaction is important for those who seek partners among friends, since almost all of the self-rating and partner-rating characteristics refer to psychological rather than physical characteristics. Such individuals describe themselves as less conventional, more intelligent, and more socially involved than those who do not seek their partners through friends. Their preferred partners are described as similarly less conventional, more socially involved, and more extroverted than the preferred partners of those who do not seek their partners through friends. These data suggest that those who seek sexual partners through friends prefer partners who are similar to themselves, and who have particular psychological characteristics. Obviously, psychological characteristics cannot be ascertained without social interaction, hence the preference, as with the previous group who contacted potential partners in bars and clubs, for social and emotional contact. In contrast with those who seek sexual partners in more anonymous settings, the emphasis is on a social relationship rather than just on sex. Those who meet partners through friends are also more masculine on the BSRI and, as expected, spend more time in the homosexual subculture (which would include homosexual social networks). They are likely to have significantly less partners per month on average over the past year, as might be expected if sexual contacts as such were less important than the individuals with whom the contacts were made.

Similarly, given that those who meet sexual partners through friends appear to place as much emphasis on social interaction as on sexual interaction, they are more likely to have had a homosexual relationship that lasted for more than two years, although less likely at present to be in a homosexual relationship that had lasted for more than two years. These data on those who contact sexual partners through friends and friendship networks suggest that there is a far greater emphasis on social rather than physical interaction in determining homosexual relationships, and that, in common with those who seek partners in bars and clubs, the emotional component of homosexual interaction is important. For those who meet partners through friends, partner numbers also decrease, which suggests that the need for sexual partners is not as driven as with more anonymous locales, and that psychological satisfaction may contribute to a lower drive for sexual partners. In general, these data from homosexual men in four countries do confirm some of the popular suppositions that suggest that individuals who seek sexual partners at less anonymous locales are more interested in the person with whom they have a sexual relationship than in simply gratifying sexual needs.

SOUTH AUSTRALIAN SAMPLE

The South Australian sample provided, as in previous chapters, an opportunity to test additional hypotheses that had been derived from the four-country sample. Data from the South Australian sample appear in Tables 8.6 to 8.10. Looking first at those individuals who make sexual contact primarily through bars and clubs, the data in Table 8.6 show that they are likely to have had much more positive parental rearing patterns than those making sexual contacts primarily in other places, with both parents having been

TABLE 8.6 Psychosocial Variables Differentiating Individuals Using Bars and Clubs as Primary Contact Point for Sexual Partners

	Not Contact Place	Contact Place
Parental rearing patterns:		
Mother rejecting	15.2	12.8*
Father overprotective	14.3	15.9*
Mother affectionate	11.6	12.9*
Father guilt-engendering	7.5	8.7*
Mother guilt-engendering	8.3	9.4+
Times STD infection past five years	1.0	2.5**
Position on Kinsey Scale past five years	5.1	5.7*
Partners per month average past year	6.0	3.7*
% sexual encounters anal insertor role	42.1	27.9*
Years homosexually active	9.0	14.7**
Alcohol days per week past five years	1.7	2.7*
Penile gonorrhea past five years	0.0	0.2**
Rectal gonorrhea past five years	0.0	0.2**
Syphilis past five years	0.0	0.1**
Penile herpes past year	0.0	0.1*
Nongonococcal urethritis past five years	0.1	0.3**

+p < .075
*p < .05
**p < .01

more accepting and affectionate. However, what does emerge is that both parents have been more guilt-engendering and the father more overprotective, which suggests overinvolvement in their son's life. It may be that meeting other homosexuals in bars and clubs serves to engender less guilt through a process of resocialization into the gay world, but the meaning of these data is far from clear. Those meeting partners in bars or clubs are more likely to be exclusively homosexual, and to have had less partners per month on average than those not preferring bars and clubs. Sexual encounters are less likely to involve the anal sex-insertor role, and as found in the four-country sample, individuals using bars and clubs are more likely to have been homosexually active for longer and thus to have presumably had more time to be socialized into homosexual institutions such as bars and clubs. Given that most bars and clubs serve alcohol, alcohol consumption levels higher than in nonbar attenders is hardly a surprise.

The role of gay bars and clubs as sexual market places is well known, and for this reason it is not surprising that bar attenders had significantly more episodes of STD infection than nonbar attenders, although they had significantly *less* partners per month on average. It is hard to understand these apparently conflicting data, unless it is assumed that bar attenders are usually recognized as attending such places specifically to pick up partners, and thus probably being more at risk of carrying or transmitting STD infection. Those infections which were elevated in incidence in bar attenders included penile gonorrhea, rectal gonorrhea, syphilis, and penile herpes as well as nongonococcal urethritis. Certainly, in terms of STD infection, bars and clubs appear to place individuals at far greater risk than other venues including saunas and cruising the beats.

Table 8.7 examines the psychosocial variables that differentiate those using cruising to contact sexual partners. Again, there is some evidence that parental rearing patterns play some part in the models of relationships one works from, with those meeting partners while cruising having parents who were overinvolved with their sons. It may be this fear of overinvolved and demanding relationships such as that with one's parents that leads those who meet partners cruising to have noninvolved and emotionally nondemanding sexual relationships. This may also explain the similar relationship in those discussed above who frequent bars. It may be that the need for a nondemanding relationship also leads individuals to seek partners in bars and clubs, but that the nature of the sexual interaction in

TABLE 8.7 Psychosocial Variables Differentiating Individuals Using Cruising Places as Primary Contact Point for Sexual Partners

	Not Contact Place	Contact Place
Parental rearing patterns:		
Mother rejecting	12.6	14.1+
Father overprotective	15.2	17.1*
Mother overprotective	15.6	17.6*
Father overinvolved	13.8	15.9*
Mother overinvolved	15.2	17.3+
Mood states:		
Anger-hostility	23.4	17.6**
Vigor	24.1	27.1+
Friendliness	20.4	23.2**
Confusion	14.9	12.2*
Depression	24.6	19.5*
Tension	20.0	16.1*
Fatigue	17.2	13.3**
Homosexual self-esteem	36.6	39.1*
Cigarettes per day past five years	1.2	2.7**
Drinks per day past five years	2.0	2.9+
Anxiety past three months[a]	4.2	3.3+

[a] 8-point scale
+p < .075
*p < .05
**p < .01

bars and clubs becomes more involved by taking place at the home of one or other of the partners, and that greater sexual contact allows for greater transmission of pathogens. This could explain the conundrum between the higher STD incidence but lower partner numbers in those frequenting bars and clubs.

Those who meet sexual partners cruising are significantly differentiated by the mood states measured by the Profile of Mood States (POMS). Cruisers are significantly less angry and hostile, less confused, less depressed, less tense and fatigued, and have more vigor and are more friendly, than noncruisers. These data strongly suggest that cruising homosexual men are more carefree and relaxed than noncruisers, and may even imply that cruising generates an euphoria, as some writers (Rechy 1963) have suggested. It is, however, impossible to separate cause from effect, and these mood states may be either the cause or the effect of cruising. It is more likely that it is a cause, since homosexual self-esteem in these individuals is higher than in noncruisers, and anxiety is lower. While cruisers drink and smoke significantly more than noncruisers, there are no other significant differences in terms of STD infections or other variables.

These data comparing cruisers with noncruisers may conflict with popular opinion, which sometimes sees cruisers as the most psychologically maladapted of the homosexual community. The data presented here suggest that the reverse is the case, and that cruisers have the most homosexual self-acceptance and the most positive mood states of the groups examined in this chapter. While this may be as a result of minimal emotional involvement, it is clear that as a sexual lifestyle it has some positive psychological concommitants.

While the data on individuals who make sexual contacts at work in the four-country study suggested that little differentiates these respondents and that they make up a small minority, we are able to investigate them further in the South Australian sample by looking at those who ranked work as a place of making sexual contacts in one of the first three categories of places of making sexual contacts, as compared with those who did not rank it at all. Table 8.8 details the psychosocial variables which differentiated the two groups. Again, the parental rearing patterns which differentiated the two groups included overprotective and overinvolved parents who were also guilt-engendering, which suggests that work as a place for sexual contacts has much in common with the locations of the sexual marketplace such as bars and clubs, and cruising. Mood states also reflected this, with the same pattern occurring as was found for cruising, namely, increased vigor and friendliness, and decreased anger-hostility and fatigue. There was increased femininity and decreased masculinity as measured on the BSRI, and on examination of individuals who reported making sexual contacts at work, most of these worked in male escort agencies, as taxi drivers, or ran homosexual establishments such as bars, clubs, or saunas. Thus for these individuals work was very similar to cruising, which explains the similar pattern of psychological variables.

There were some marked differences, however, on variables relating to risk factors. Those meeting sexual contacts at work had a markedly higher number of STD infections in the past five years, as well as significantly

TABLE 8.8 Psychosocial Variables Differentiating Individuals Using
Work as Primary Contact Point for Sexual Partners

	Not Contact Place	Contact Place
Parental rearing patterns:		
Father overprotective	15.2	16.7+
Mother overprotective	15.8	17.9*
Mother overinvolved	15.1	17.5+
Father guilt-engendering	8.1	9.2+
Mother guilt-engendering	8.7	10.5*
Father favors respondent	6.3	8.1*
Mood states:		
Anger-hostility	21.5	16.9**
Vigor	25.2	28.4*
Friendliness	21.7	23.8*
Fatigue	16.1	13.9*
Masculinity	12.1	9.5*
Femininity	14.4	18.3**
Times STD infection past five years	1.7	4.1*
Partners per month average past year	3.8	4.6+
% sexual encounters fellatio	69.1	81.7*
% sexual encounters analingus	18.6	35.8*
Pharangeal gonorrhea past five years	0.1	0.0+

+p < .075
*p < .05
**p < .01

more partners per month average. They had significantly
higher percentages of fellatio and analingus compared with
those who did not meet partners at work, but had had
pharyngeal gonorrhea less often than the comparison group.
Taken together, those data confirm that psychologically,
this group has much in common with the cruising group,
but also have significantly higher partner numbers and STD
infections. Essentially, such individuals are cruisers who
are by reason of occupation exposed to constant cruising,
and hence the marked increase in partners and STD infections. They are, however, still numerically a small group,
numbering only about 10 percent of the sample.

There appear to be few variables in the South Australian sample which differentiate between those who make
sexual contacts primarily through friends and those who do

TABLE 8.9 Psychosocial Variables Differentiating Individuals Making Sexual Contact through Friends

	No Contact	Contact
Mood states:		
Vigor	25.2	27.8+
% leisure time spent in homosexual subculture	38.9	50.0*
% sexual encounters sadomasochistic	10.5	0.0**
Cigarettes per day past year	19	10.0*

+p < .075
*p < .05
**p < .01

not. Those variables that do discriminate appear in Table 8.9: no parental rearing patterns are implicated. In terms of mood states, vigor is higher in those meeting partners through friends, and as anticipated a greater proportion of leisure time is spent in the homosexual subculture (of which gay friendship networks is a part). None of those making sexual contact through friends had sadomasochistic encounters, and they also tended to smoke less. Clearly, there is little that can be said about those who make sexual contacts through friends from these meager data.

This cannot be said for the data on those who make their sexual contacts primarily at saunas and bath houses. Table 8.10 illustrates the variables which discriminate the two groups of those who do and who do not make contacts at the gay sauna in South Australia, and it is immediately clear that parental rearing patterns are one of the major discriminators. Those using the sauna for sexual contact have much more negative paternal and maternal rearing patterns, with parents who, in addition, were overinvolved, overprotective and performance-oriented. This pattern does suggest that casual and nonemotionally involving sexual contacts, at least in this venue, have abusive, depriving, punitive, and shaming parents as a concomitant and that this may lead to a rejection of, or inability to, relate emotionally to others. Sexual contacts in bath houses may also act as a means of reducing anxiety and increasing self-esteem that has been created by negative and overinvolved parents. It is of particular interest that the patterns of individuals who make their sexual contacts cruising and those who make them in bath houses are radically different

TABLE 8.10 Psychosocial Variables Differentiating Individuals Making
Sexual Contact at Saunas

	No Contact	Contact
Parental rearing patterns:		
Father abusive	8.5	10.0*
Father depriving	9.5	11.3*
Mother depriving	9.3	10.8**
Father punitive	12.5	15.4*
Mother punitive	12.3	14.0*
Father shaming	7.3	8.8*
Mother overprotective	15.7	17.6*
Father overinvolved	13.9	15.8+
Mother overinvolved	14.7	17.6*
Mother affectionate	12.9	11.5*
Father performance-oriented	11.4	13.4**
Mother performance-oriented	12.4	13.7+
Father guilt-engendering	7.8	9.1*
Father favors respondent	7.6	5.8**
Mood states:		
Depression[a]	18.7	21.6*
Symptoms of illness	0.6	1.8**
Marijuana use days per month past year	1.3	3.0*
Marijuana use days per month past five years	1.7	3.6*
Depressed past three months[a]	1.9	2.9**
Penile gonorrhea past five years	0.1	0.4**
Anorectal warts past five years	0.2	0.1*
Nongonococcal urethritis past five years	0.4	0.2*

[a] 8-point scale
+p < .075
*p < .05
**p < .01

apart from the common element of overinvolved parents, and
that despite the apparent similarity of brief sexual contacts,
usually without emotional content, the two are markedly
different. Cruising also involves more one-to-one contact
and will usually be a single contact, while bath houses may
provide for multiple noninvolved contacts.

Those making sexual contacts primarily in bath houses
are also more depressed both in terms of the POMS and the
visual analog scale, measuring depression that suggests
strongly that negative mood states are related to multiple

anonymous contacts, and that such contacts may serve to decrease depression or at least hold it in check. Depression may also most probably make any level of meaningful emotional contact difficult. Those using the sauna for sexual contacts also report increased use of marijuana, and while they do not appear to have significantly increased numbers of sexual partners or STD infections, they are more likely to have had penile gonorrhea and less likely to have had anorectal warts or nongonococcal urethritis. One can therefore conclude that while this is a small sample, there are distinct differences between the determinants of each of the modes and venues of primary sexual contacts. The negative influences, both in terms of mood states and parental rearing patterns, are clear in the case of bath house contacts but quite dissimilar to other places of casual contact. However, the negative associations of increased partner numbers and increased STD infections in the sauna sample are not at all evident.

In conclusion, these data taken together do demonstrate some marked differences between those preferring particular places of meeting sexual partners. Those meeting in bars tend to prefer social as well as emotional contacts but had overinvolved parents that may have made extended interaction difficult, and those making contacts through friends prefer homosocial as well as homosexual contacts to an even greater degree. Contrary to expectations, those meeting partners through cruising have more positive mood states and higher self-esteem than others, and were markedly different to those who frequented saunas. These latter individuals appear to be more depressed and more avoiding of close emotional contacts, probably as a result of much more negative parental rearing practices experienced, which may have provided negative relationship models.

These findings again cast some light on the potential dynamics of those involved in meeting partners at particular venues, and particularly in terms of those who attend homosexual bath houses. They also suggest potential interventions that might be available to decrease the attendance at such locales or at least to ensure that sexual contacts do not maintain the driven quality that appears to be associated with sexual contacts in saunas. Again, an understanding of the psychosocial factors that are associated with partner contact may offer some solutions for moves to lower-risk behavior patterns.

9

Attitudes Toward Sexuality and Their Relationship to Sexual Behavior

While it has been possible to discover a number of psychological and social variables that are associated with specific risk factors such as increased partner numbers, particular sexual activities, and frequenting certain locales for sexual contact, such information in itself is not entirely adequate to attempt to understand or modify such behaviors. If we are to assume in addition that particular attitudes toward sexuality underlie sexual behaviors in general, we must attempt to measure and understand such sexual behaviors and to determine whether they do in fact underlie specific sexual behaviors. However, Eysenck (1976) has commented that "Obviously sexual behaviour is so complex, and determined by so many factors, both systematic and accidental, that no single factor could account for a very large proportion of the variance." Clearly, it may in practice be difficult to measure and describe sexual attitudes and expect much reliability.

Eysenck factor-analyzed the responses of 423 male and 379 female university students to 98 questions that covered a range of attitudes to sexuality, and found that oblique rotation yielded thirteen interpretable factors. These covered the domains of sexual satisfaction, sexual excitement, sexual nervousness, sexual curiosity, attitudes to premarital sex, sexual repression, prudishness, sexual experimentation, attitudes toward homosexuality, attitudes toward censorship, attitudes toward promiscuity, sexual hostility, and sexual guilt. These factors occurred with both males and females, and appeared to be stable in structure in both samples. Subsequently, Eysenck investigated sexual attitudes in 427 male and 436 female adults with an average age of around 30 years, using the same questionnaire expanded by 60 questions to 158 items. Oblique factor analysis of 135 of these items produced over 40 dimensions with eigenvalues greater than unity, but 12 factors were interpretable. These 12 factors covered the following attitudinal areas: permissiveness, satisfaction, neurotic sex, impersonal sex, pornography, sexual shyness, prudishness, dominance-submission, sexual disgust, sexual excitement, physical sex, and aggressive sex. Factor comparison coefficients between the male and female factor solutions were all highly significant (ranging from .52 to .97, median .89), confirming that the factor structure was again stable between the sexes.

The reliability and the large range of interpretable dimensions achieved by Eysenck (1976) raises a number of questions as the their applicability to sexual, and particularly homosexual, behavior. Eysenck, in his initial study on the sexual attitudes of university students, found that high psychoticism scorers also tended to score higher on sexual curiosity, attitudes to premarital sex, promiscuity, and hostility scales, being more sexually curious, more accepting of premarital sex, more promiscuous, and more hostile. Extroverts tended to score high on the promiscuity scales and low on the nervousness scale (more promiscuous and less sexually nervous), while high scorers on the neuroticism scale had significantly lower scores on sexual satisfaction, and significantly higher scores on excitement, nervousness, sexual hostility, sexual guilt, and sexual inhibition. As well as having high construct validity, these results fit in surprisingly well with those of Hart (1973b, c). Hart found that extroversion was a marked feature of those with STD infection in his study of Australian soldiers in Vietnam, and that high neuroticism scores were closely associated with venereoneurosis. Clearly, Hart's data, along with those of Wells (1969), parallel those of Eysenck (1976) in the finding of a close association between extroversion and STD infections. Hart went so far as to comment (Hart 1973b) that "certain sociological parameters to venereal infection may be of a secondary nature, in that all are primarily related to the personality of the individual."

More recently, Fulford et al. (1983b) used Eysenck's personality measures of psychoticism, extroversion, neuroticism, and their associated Lie scale (Eysenck and Eysenck 1975) and found that while neuroticism correlated positively

with syphilis and gonorrhea infections, extroversion correlated negatively with the diagnosis of syphilis. These
findings are somewhat confusing and in the opposite direction to what might be expected from previous research.
However, Fulford et al. (1983b) also used the second
(adult) versions of Eysenck's (1976) sexual attitudes questionnaire in the sample of 180 male STD clinic attenders,
and found that their total samples scored lower than
Eysenck's adult male sample on the factors measuring interest in pornography, sexual excitement, interest in physical
sex, interest in aggressive sex, and displayed greater
prudishness and sexual disgust. These results are also in
the opposite direction to that expected. The only difference between small subsamples of heterosexual and homosexual men was that homosexual clinic attenders had a lower
interest in physical sex, again contrary to what might be
expected. Bisexual men, however, scored significantly
higher than heterosexuals for neurotic sex, impersonal sex,
prudishness, and sexual disgust, and lower on sexual
excitement, which suggests that their bisexual respondents
had atypically abnormal sexual attitudes. Fulford et al.
report that the differences between the total clinic sample
and Eysenck's adult sample were mainly due to the contribution of the bisexual men. They did not, however, examine the links between the sexual attitudes in the sample and
STD infections. Given that their respondents were all from
an STD clinic, the lack of significant differences between
their sample and Eysenck's adult males (apart from the
differences that were contributed to by the bisexual males)
suggests that sexual attitudes played little part in determining STD infection.

However, examination of Eysenck's (1976) 158-item
sexual attitudes questionnaire reveals that many of the
questions are inappropriate for homosexual men, since the
test was designed with a heterosexual majority in mind
(apart from a number of questions designed to detect a
homoerotic orientation). It is probable, therefore, that the
comparison of scale scores between homosexuals and heterosexuals by Fulford et al. (1983b) was marred by items that
would have been meaningless to homosexual men. If we are
to test the hypothesis that sexual attitudes are an important
underlying dimension of sexual behaviors, particularly those
associated with STD infections, then it is important to
establish first whether Eysenck's sexual attitudes questionnaire can be modified to make it appropriate for homosexuals, and second, whether such a modified questionnaire
produces the same factors in homosexuals as in heterosexual
men and women.

REASONS FOR DIFFERENCES IN SEXUAL ATTITUDES BETWEEN HOMOSEXUALS AND HETEROSEXUALS

There are several reasons why a form of Eysenck's sexual attitudes questionnaire may not provide the same dimensions in homosexuals as in heterosexuals. First, because the meaning of sexuality to homosexuals is quite different to the meaning of sexuality to heterosexuals. Despite major advances in contraception in the past few decades (and particularly the widespread use of the anovulent pill), sex and reproduction are closely linked in the heterosexual consciousness, and in many cases when heterosexuals are asked the purpose of sexuality, their response is usually explicitly or implicitly linked to child bearing and child raising. In contrast, to the homosexual male the meaning of sexuality is more likely to be related to hedonistic factors or to expressions of emotional closeness, and the communicative aspect of sexuality emphasized. While relating sexuality to reproduction, it must be noted that the presence of children may radically alter interpersonal and sexual relationships since the children, rather than the partner, often become the focus of the household. However, this is not necessarily limited to heterosexuals, since there may be many childless couples and since homosexuals may also have children.

A second factor that may lead to major differences in sexuality between homosexual and heterosexual men relates to models of sexual behavior promoted by Western society, and the socialization of individuals into heterosexual or homosexual models. While it has been observed frequently enough previously that homosexuals are born into heterosexual relationships, when the individual identifies himself as a homosexual, a certain and variable amount of the heterosexual model is rejected. In some cases, the total rejection of the heterosexual model will lead to sexual attitudes that emphasize equality of partners, role rejection, and rejection of long-term or monogamous interactions. For individuals whose sexual attitudes fall into this latter group, sexual attitudes can be expected to differ markedly from those of most heterosexuals, since what homosexuality is seen as providing is an alternative model of relating to other humans, and sexual behavior is seen as a subset of this alternative model. To the extent that homosexuality is seen as different both qualitatively and quantitatively from heterosexuality, the sexual attitudes and sexual behaviors of the individual may also be expected to differ.

Third, attitudes toward sexuality are frequently an implicit part of religious beliefs, although even within such religious systems as Christianity and Judaism there are multiple shades of interpretation. Insofar as most Western societies are explicitly or implicitly "Christian" societies, there is usually an undercurrent of rejection of homosexual behaviors, particularly between males. Since homosexuals may be seen as outcasts, and as rejectors of (and rejected by) the Judeo-Christian teachings, many homosexuals may have thus rejected religious and social mores as inapplicable to them. Freed of conventional morality by their rejection of it, homosexuals are thus to greater or lesser extent freed of the conventional mores relating to sexual behavior and thus sexual attitudes. To a greater degree than most heterosexuals, then, they are in a position to form their own attitudes and to be socialized anew in the homosexual subculture, which has its own norms and morality in many way distinct from those of most heterosexuals. For this reason I believe that the era of socialization into a homosexual subculture, the nature of that subculture, and the age at which it occurs are likely to be critical determinants of the attitudes to sexuality and homosexuality of the individual.

As a further extension of this point, the very act of having to question current sexual attitudes and mores performs the function of rejecting some, rationalizing others, or redefining old attitudes in terms of situational ethics, and adapting them to a new sexual lifestyle. This questioning and redefinition of previously unquestional attitudes to sexuality will be familiar to most sexologists, and to a degree occurs in most homosexuals as they realize the extent to which homosexual behavior is stigmatized in Western society.

Realization that one's sexuality is stigmatized will in itself lead to a degree of redefinition of sexual attitudes. Such a realization leads to an inevitable redefinition of self, and if the negative societal attitudes to homosexuality are maintained, the consequence is lowered self-esteem and acceptance of a deviant status. The consequences of public labeling may be even more important in the formation of sexual attitudes, and in this regard societal reaction to homosexuality is a variable that cannot be dismissed in terms of its subsequent influence on the psychological development of the homosexual (Ross 1985e). Homosexual men who see themselves as religious outcasts, psychologically unstable, or doomed to lonely or furtive sexual interactions will have totally different sexual attitudes to those who accept their sexuality, and the dimension of attitudes to homosexuality will more probably approximate that of heterosexual sample in the former. While to a large extent these hypotheses will need to be empirically tested, the effect of societal reaction and societal stigma on the functioning of the homosexual man will almost certainly have a major influence on his sexual attitudes and probably, if we believe that attitudes underlie behavior, on his sexual functioning. The importance, therefore, of sexual attitudes to venereology is obvious but is still far from being sufficiently obvious.

One final factor that may affect sexual attitudes and create differences in these attitudes between homosexuals and heterosexuals is the fact that by definition homosexual relationships occur between members of the same gender, and heterosexual relationships between members of opposite genders. In terms of its meaning for sexual attitudes, this has two profound influences. First, it leads to a far greater understanding and appreciation of the sexual partner in a homosexual relationship, in which one is dealing with an individual who is far better understood in terms of physiological response and sexual reaction by being of the same gender. One is reminded of the comment that in the 1950s, sex was something men did *to* women. In the 1960s, it was something they did *for* women. In the 1970s, it was something they did *with* women. In the 1980s, and for the homosexual since homosexual relations existed, it was not necessary for a male to have sex with a *woman*. For the homosexual man, therefore, sex was more able to be understood in terms of his own needs and feelings without the barriers of different social roles, physiological reactions, different sexual apparatus, and in many cases differences in dominance as a result of differential social statuses for males and females. This second fact, that of different social status, may occur in homosexual relationships across class, socioeconomic, or educational or cultural divides, but does not alter the conclusion that a homosexual relationship provides an interaction that is one of likes rather than dislikes. In this regard, a homosexual relationship may engender a more empathic understanding of a partner (at least in sexual terms), and the effects of this on sexual attitudes may be to emphasize the emotional and empathic nature of homosexual and homosocial relationships on the one hand, and sexual on the other. Given that, at least in Western society, the double standard still exists to an extent, and it is seen as more acceptable for males to indulge in sexual contacts than it is for females, there is a multiplicative effect of this double standard when a sexual interaction is between two males. The effect of this on sexual attitudes cannot be calculated, but it may have the effect of removing sex role considerations from attitudes to sexuality as well as removing questions about partner numbers, monogamy, and sexual practices from the position of relative importance they occupy in Eysenck's (1976) factor solution.

Many of these questions raised above as to the source of potential differences between sexual attitudes of homosexual and heterosexual men, however, beg the question of whether in practice such differences do exist. It could be argued that the lack of major differences in factor structure between the males and females in Eysenck's sample suggest the opposite argument: namely, that sexual attitudes are relatively stable across the genders, and that there is every reason to believe that they will be fairly equivalent across homosexual and heterosexual samples. This basic question must be answered before we are able to pose, and answer, the second question as to whether sexual attitudes affect or underlie the sexual behaviors that lead to increased risk of STD infection.

SAMPLE AND METHOD

The study reported in this chapter used two samples of homosexual men. The first, the South Australian sample, was identical to the South Australian sample reported in Chapter 3, but with the addition of a further 90 homosexual men who were surveyed in two public meetings in Adelaide, South Australia. The first meeting was a forum on AIDS, the second the annual meeting of a homosexual social and counseling organization. The mean age of respondents for this total sample of 187 South Australian homosexual men was 33.7±8.6 years.

The second sample, the Californian sample, was collected in the Bay area of San Francisco, and numbered 179 homosexual men. This sample was recruited in two ways: by asking homosexual men attending two predominantly gay medical practices in San Francisco to complete the questionnaire in the waiting room prior to consultation, and by asking homosexual men who were interviewed by the author as part of a separate study in San Francisco to also complete questionnaires. The mean age of the San Francisco sample was 31.9±9.3 years.

The questionnaire (Appendix 4) was derived from that used by Eysenck (1976) for his adult male and female sample. Eysenck's questionnaire, 158 items long, was truncated in three ways. First, items that appeared to be heterosexually biased or relevant only to heterosexual interactions were excluded. Examples of such questions include the following: "Sex should be used for the purpose of reproduction, not for personal pleasure" (Q.88); "Females do hot have such a strong sex desire as males" (Q.94); "One should not experiment with sex before marriage"(Q.38); "Virginity is a girl's most valuable possession" (Q.5); and "The idea of 'wife-swapping' is extremely distasteful to me" (Q.135).

Second, those questions that referred to attitudes toward homosexuality were deleted, since it did not seem reasonable to alter them to provide a scale of attitudes toward heterosexuality. Examples of questions deleted include: "I love physical contact with members of my own sex" (Q.138); "Frankly, I prefer people of my own sex" (Q.15); "I understand homosexuals" (Q.36); and "People of my own sex frequently attract me" (Q.33). There seemed little sense in attempting to thus identify homosexuals in a homosexual sample!

Third, all those questions that did not load above 0.3 on the 12 male factors that Eysenck derived from his adult male sample were deleted. Finally, all those questions that referred to opposite-gender partners were changed to refer to same-gender partners. This final form of the questionnaire, 89 items in total, is illustrated in Appendix 4.

Statistical analysis consisted of separate analysis of the South Australian and Californian data. Both data sets were subject to initial principal components analysis and then subject to oblique rotation (direct oblimin), with the delta level set a zero to ensure a correlated solution. Initial analysis of the South Australian data revealed 30 factors with eigenvalues greater than unity, so the analysis was carried out a second time limiting the number of factors to nine (the number of dimensions with eigenvalues greater than two). These nine dimensions were all interpretable and those items which had loadings of greater than 0.4 are illustrated in Table 9.1.

In the case of the Californian data, initial factor analysis followed the same pattern as in the South Australian data, and the 11 factors with eigenvalues greater than two subject to similar oblique rotation. However, because of the small number of items loading above 0.4 in some of the factors extracted last, the loading for inclusion was set at greater than 0.35. The factor pattern of the Californian data is illustrated in Table 9.2.

Since the South Australian data were obtained in conjunction with other data on STD infections, sexual practices, partner numbers, and preferred places of sexual contact, the obtained dimensions of sexual attitudes were factor-scored by multiplying the item score ($A=1$, $?=2$, $D=3$)

by the factor loading, and multiplying by 10 to obtain manageable figures. The resulting factor scores are thus able to be illustrated in relation to these other data, and appear in Tables 9.3, 9.4, and 9.5. Since the Californian data were obtained only to provide an estimate of whether there was stability of sexual attitudes of homosexual men across cultures, they were not collected with any data relating to STD risk factors and consequently not factor-scored.

RESULTS AND DISCUSSION

The point must be strongly made at the beginning of discussion of the results that this study was exploratory, and that the numbers of respondents necessary for carrying out factor analyses was therefore at the lower limit of what is statistically advisable. It must further be made clear that the truncation of Eysenck's questionnaire, while carried out to maximize the possibility of comparable results to those obtained from his adult male sample, may have nevertheless introduced some systematic bias (for example, by excluding questions relating to attitudes to heterosexual sex and to females). However, these are questions that must be addressed in subsequent research on the dimensionality of sexual attitudes in homosexual men, and we shall not concern ourselves with them further in the analysis of these data.

SOUTH AUSTRALIAN ATTITUDES

As illustrated in Table 9.1, nine interpretable dimensions were extracted for the South Australian homosexual men. These were labeled, in order of extraction, Fear of Sexual Relationships, Interest in Pornography, Sexual Excitability, Comfort with Women, Acceptance of Sexuality, Importance of Affect and Relationships, Prudishness, General Permissiveness, and Libido and Sexual Control.

Factor 1 (Fear of Sexual Relationships) is characterized by items that suggest that this dimension is tapping a guilt-ridden concern about sexual relationships, dissatisfaction with one's sex life, and intrusive thoughts about sex. It contains five items from Eysenck's Satisfaction factor and the five further items from his Neurotic Sex factor (these factors are in fact correlated -.31 in the adult male sample on which he reports). However, it is apparent that the combination expresses something that is quite different in

TABLE 9.1 Factor Sturcture of Sexual Attitudes Inventory in Australian
Homosexual Men

FACTOR 1: Fear of Sexual Relationships

75	I am afraid of sexual relationships.	.80
71	I feel sexually less competent than my friends.	.79
36	Sometimes thinking about sex makes me very nervous.	.70
25	My conscience bothers me too much.	.66
18	My parent's influence has inhibited me sexually.	.64
19	Thoughts about sex disturb me more than they should.	.63
3	All in all I am satisfied with my sex life.	-.61
11	Something is lacking in my sex life.	.57
43	I have been involved with more than one sex affair at the same time.	-.54
7	I have been deprived sexually.	.53
34	I worry a lot about sex.	.47
14	I have felt guilty about sex experiences.	.44
44	I have sometimes felt hostile to my sex partner.	.43

(17.8% of variance)

FACTOR 2: Interest in Pornography

46	If I had the chance to see people making love, without being seen, I would take it.	.82
73	The thought of an illicit relationship excites me.	.69
45	I like to look at pictures of nudes.	.59
87	If you were offered a highly pornographic book, would you accept it? (yes)	.53
24	I like to look at sexy pictures.	.53
66	Most men are sex-mad.	.46
72	Group sex appeals to me.	.45
77	Physical sex is the most important part of marriage.	.43
70	I sometimes feel like scratching and biting my partner during intercourse.	.42
12	My sex behavior has never caused me any trouble.	-.42

(17.5% of variance)

FACTOR 3: Sexual Excitement

17	It doesn't take much to get me sexually excited.	.79
2	Conditions have to be just right to get me excited sexually.	-.71
42	I have sometimes felt like humiliating my sex partner.	.56
74	I usually feel aggressive with my sexual partner.	.56
21	I get excited sexually very easily.	.49
89	Have you ever suffered from impotence? (no)	.48
40	I believe in taking my pleasures where I find them.	.41

(12.0% of variance)

FACTOR 4: Comfort with Women

30	I feel at ease with people of the opposite sex.	-.75
9	It is disturbing to see necking in public.	.55
27	I feel nervous with the opposite sex.	.54
81	I object to four-letter swear words being used in mixed company.	.49

TABLE 9.1   Continued

39	Sex jokes disgust me.	.48
13	My love-life has been disappointing.	.46
34	I worry a lot about sex.	-.45
	(10.5% of variance)	

FACTOR 5: Acceptance of Sexuality

16	I have strong sex feelings but when I get a chance I can't seem to express myself.	-.60
6	I get pleasant feelings from touching my sexual parts.	-.52
52	Sex is far and away my greatest pleasure.	-.52
53	Sexual permissiveness threatens to undermine the entire foundation of civilized society.	-.48
29	When I get excited I can think of nothing else but satisfaction.	-.47
67	Being good in bed is terribly important to my partner.	-.47
	(8.0% of variance)	

FACTOR 6: Importance of Affect and Relationship

79	In a sexual union, tenderness is the most important quality.	.61
84	It would not disturb me over much if my sexual partner had sexual relations with someone else, as long as he returned to me.	-.60
64	My sex partner satisfies all my physical needs completely.	.55
58	I prefer partners who are several years older than myself.	.43
67	Being good in bed is terribly important to my partner.	.42
	(7.9% of variance)	

FACTOR 7: Prudishness

83	The naked human body is a pleasing sight.	.55
9	It is disturbing to see necking in public.	-.52
69	I would like my sex partner to be more expert and experienced.	.45
49	There are too many immoral plays on TV.	.44
35	Seeing a person nude doesn't interest me.	-.42
	(7.5% of variance)	

FACTOR 8: Permissiveness

56	Sex play among children is quite harmless.	-.71
48	Prostitution should be legally permitted.	-.57
22	The thought of a sex orgy is disgusting to me.	.54
77	Physical sex is the most important part of marriage.	.42
53	Sexual permissiveness threatens to undermine the entire foundation of civilized society.	.42
50	I had some bad sex experiences when I was young.	.41
	(6.6% of variance)	

FACTOR 9: Libido and Control

28	Sex thoughts drive me almost crazy.	.68
72	Group sex appeals to me.	.45
26	Sometimes sexual feelings overpower me.	.41
29	When I get excited I can think of nothing else but satisfaction.	.41
	(6.3% of variance)	

concept from Eysenck's two factors for heterosexuals, since it captures the guilt and self-doubt that leads to avoidance of sex and sexual relationships. While this could occur in a similar form in heterosexuals, it does appear more typical of the effects of stigma and societal rejection of a homosexual lifestyle and probably should be interpreted in this manner.

Factor 2 (Interest in Pornography) is a fairly coherent factor that contains clusters of items indicating both an interest in pornography and an associated affirmation that need for physical sex is an important part of the male personality. While it contains four items from Eysenck's Pornography factor, it also contains two items from his Permissiveness scale, and appears to tap not only a voyeuristic dimension but also an associated set of beliefs and behaviors about an increased interest in physical sex and sexual affairs. Here, there appears to be a nexus between visual stimulation and physical interest in sex. Again, this is not a pure factor as was Eysenck's Pornography factor, but an indication that in homosexual men, visual stimulation is associated with sexual arousal.

Factor 3 (Sexual Excitement) is substantially similar to that of Eysenck, containing four of the five items of his scale. It also contains items that associate aggressive sex with sexual excitement. These two factors have a correlation of only .08 in Eysenck's adult male sample, so it could be the case that the linking of sexual excitement and aggressive sex is more common in homosexual than in heterosexual men.

Factor 4 (Comfort with Women) contains items that suggest both discomfort with women and lack of permissiveness, with two items from Eysenck's Shyness scale and the same number from his Permissiveness scale. The combination is unusual, and is probably peculiar to homosexual men who are uncomfortable both with females and with gender-inappropriate behavior like sex jokes and swearwords in mixed company. This discomfort with women would appear to be based on sex role conservatism and a belief in different socially appropriate behaviors in the presence of males and females.

Factor 5 (Acceptance of Sexuality) has three items from Eysenck's Physical Sex factor loading significantly on it, but combines acceptance of one's sexual feelings with items expressing acceptance of genital pleasure and the importance of being sexually competent. While this factor has connotations of interest in physical sex in heterosexual men, its interpretation in homosexual men would appear to suggest an acceptance of their homosexual feelings and positive feelings about them. It also suggests a degree of hedonism, which would be expected to be associated with acceptance of physical sex.

Factor 6 (Importance of Affect and Relationship) again has little correspondence with any of the factors Eysenck found in his adult heterosexual sample, but is readily interpretable in terms of a homosexual sample. This factor defines the dimension of the importance of affect in relationships, of monogamy, the ability to have one partner satisfy all needs, and again the importance of the sexual side of a relationship. The importance of this factor in measuring affective and relational aspects of á homosexual lifestyle should not be underestimated, since it expresses attitudes that are often taken for granted in a heterosexual context but are unusual in some homosexual contexts.

Factor 7 (Prudishness) in fact is an amalgam of Eysenck's Prudishness and Permissiveness factors, although it does not contain many items. It expresses concerns about nudity and public aspects of morality and can probably best be described in terms of prudishness. Factor 8 (Permissiveness) is essentially similar to Eysenck's Permissiveness factor, and although it contains only six items, four of these are from Eysenck's Permissiveness scale. There appears to be no reason why it should not be interpreted in much the same way as Eysenck interpreted it.

Factor 9 (Libido and Control) does contain two items from Eysenck's Physical Sex dimension, but the consistency of its items, all of which relate to control of strong libido, make its interpretation easy. It is clear that it relates to control of sexual impulses rather than the presence of these, and for this reason is taken as measuring a dimension that has no parallel to any of those derived by Eysenck.

In general, then, there is a degree of correspondence between the factors derived by Eysenck from his adult males and those derived from the South Australian sample of homosexual men. However, when examined in closer detail, it is apparent that many of the homosexual attitudinal dimensions have different meanings from the heterosexual ones and that the mix of items conveys a different flavor. For this reason, it would appear that the dimensionality of sexual attitudes in South Australian homosexual men is sufficiently different from the dimensionality of attitudes in Eysenck's (1976) adult heterosexual male sample to justify using separate dimensions.

A second point worthy of note is that less than 60 of the 89 items of the revised questionnaire loaded significantly on the nine interpretable factors, suggesting that many of the items in Eysenck's original questionnaire are of little relevance or have little discriminating power in a homosexual sample. However, it is probably most important to assess the same 89-item questionnaire used on the South Australian homosexual men on a further homosexual sample in order to assess its stability across samples.

CALIFORNIAN ATTITUDES

In contrast to the sexual attitudes of South Australian homosexual men, the factor structure of the Californian homosexual men produced 11 factors, none of which accounted for more than 9 percent of variance. These factors are illustrated in Table 9.2. The dimensions which appear in Table 9.2 bear little relationship to either the factor structures obtained by Eysenck (1976) or in the South Australian homosexual sample.

Factor 1 (Lack of Monogamy) contains three items from Eysenck's Sexual Excitement factor, but the other items make it clear that this is to be specifically interpreted as acceptance of nonmonogamous relationships. This particular factor is in marked contrast to the Importance of Affect and Relationship factor in the South Australian men. Factor 2 (Libido and Control) does have three items in common with the South Australian factor of the same name, and appears to tap the same dimension, although emphasizing also the hedonistic aspect of sex. Factor 3 (Permissiveness) contains three items that also figure in Eysenck's Permissiveness scale, although it contains only one item in common with the South Australian Permissiveness scale. Factor 4 (Interest in Pornography), while again tapping much the same dimensions as Eysenck's Pornography factor, with which it has four items in common, has three items in common with the South Australian factor of the same name. It seems reasonable to conclude that this dimension is the same in all three samples.

Factor 5 (Unnamed) is difficult to interpret, and contains two items from Eysenck's Permissiveness scale. Factor 6 (Comfort with Women) has two items in common with the scale of the same name in the South Australian factor solution, but does not contain the connotations of sex-role rigidity as it does in that scale. Also unnamed, Factor 7 is as difficult to interpret as Factor 5, but contains the implication of a negative cognitive dimension. However, the juxtaposition of items makes little intuitive sense. Factor 8 (Prudishness), while probably containing too few items for adequate interpretation, does suggest a coherent dislike of the overtly sexual.

TABLE 9.2 Factor Structure of Sexual Attitudes Inventory in American Homosexual Men

---

FACTOR 1: Lack of Monogamy

84	It would not disturb me over much if my sex partner had sexual relations with someone else, as long as he returned to me.	.64
54	Absolute faithfulness to one partner throughout life is nearly as silly as celibacy.	.60
17	It doesn't take much to get me excited sexually.	.53
21	I get excited sexually very easily.	.53
55	I would enjoy watching my usual partner having intercourse with someone else.	.50
2	Conditions have to be just right to get me excited sexually.	-.49
10	Sexual feelings are sometimes unpleasant to me.	-.43
72	Group sex appeals to me.	.39

(8.8% of variance)

FACTOR 2: Libido and Control

26	Sometimes sexual feelings overpower me.	.70
52	Sex is far and away my greatest pleasure.	.60
15	At times I have been afraid of myself for what I might do sexually.	.60
28	Sex thoughts drive me almost crazy.	.57
29	When I get excited I can think of nothing else but satisfaction.	.56
63	To me few things are more important than sex.	.53
4	Sometimes it Has been a problem to control my sex feelings.	.45
23	I find the thought of a colored sex partner particularly exiting.	.45
66	Most men are sex mad.	.39
19	Thoughts about sex disturb me more than they should.	.36

(6.2% of variance)

FACTOR 3: Permissiveness

47	Pornographic writings should be freely allowed to be published.	-.62
51	There should be no censorship, on sexual grounds, of plays and films.	-.58
64	My sex partner satisfies all my physical needs completely.	.56
83	The naked human body is a pleasing sight.	-.50
53	Sexual permissiveness threatens to undermine the entire foundation of civilized society.	.38
27	I feel nervous with the opposite sex.	.38
16	I have strong sex feelings but when I get the chance I can't seem to express myself.	.37

(5.3% of variance)

FACTOR 4: Interest in Pornography

24	I like to look at sexy pictures.	-.83
45	I like to look at pictures of nudes.	-.73
35	Seeing a person nude doesn't interest me.	.63
46	If I had the chance to see people making love, without being seen, I would take it.	-.56
21	I get excited sexually very easily.	-.37

(4.7% of variance)

TABLE 9.2 Continued

FACTOR 5: Unnamed

42	I have sometimes felt like humiliating my sex partner.	.61
48	Prostitution should be legally permitted.	.36
56	Sex play among children is quite harmless.	.35
10	Sexual feelings are sometimes unpleasant to me.	.35

(3.9% of variance)

FACTOR 6: Comfort with Women

30	I feel at ease with people of the opposite sex.	-.67
27	I feel nervous with the opposite sex.	.52
69	I would like my sex partner to be more expert and experienced.	.47
32	It is hard to talk with people of the opposite sex.	.44

(3.7% of variance)

FACTOR 7: Unnamed

37	Perverted sex thoughts have sometimes bothered me.	.68
36	Sometimes thinking about sex makes me very nervous.	.45
77	Physical sex is the most important part of marriage.	.45
33	I enjoy petting.	.40

(3.6% of variance)

FACTOR 8: Prudishness

80	Male genitals are aesthetically unpleasing.	-.62
39	Sex jokes disgust me.	-.56
49	There are too many immoral plays on TV.	-.40

(3.4% of variance)

FACTOR 9: Sexual Inhibitions

82	I cannot discuss sexual matters with my habitual sex partner.	.66
76	I can't stand people touching me.	.62
85	Some forms of love-making are disgusting to me.	.58
31	I don't like to be kissed.	.36

(3.6% of variance)

FACTOR 10: Importance of Sexual Attractiveness and Competence

9	It is disturbing to see necking in public.	.53
78	Physical attraction is extremely important to me.	-.52
67	Being good in bed is terribly important to my partner.	-.42
40	I believe in taking my pleasures where I find them.	-.35

(3.0% of variance)

FACTOR 11: Fear of Sexual Relationships

71	I feel sexually less competent than my friends.	.64
7	I have been deprived sexually.	.63
8	Sex contacts have never been a problem to me.	-.60
25	My conscience bothers me too much.	.49
68	I find it easy to tell my sex partner what I like, or don't like, about his lovemaking.	-.47
16	I have strong sex feelings but when I get the chance I can't seem to express myself.	.38
13	My love life has been disappointing.	

(2.8% of variance)

Factor 9 (Sexual Inhibitions) is consistent and refers to inhibitions about sexual discussion and physical sexual contact, and corresponds neither with a South Australian factor nor with one of Eysenck's factors. Factor 10 (Importance of Sexual Attractiveness and Competence) is again difficult to interpret, but appears to draw together a need to maintain self-esteem in a sexual context. Finally, Factor 11 (Fear of Sexual Relationships) does contain three items in common with the factor of the same name in the South Australian factor structure, but the remaining items convey a feeling more of sexual inhibition than of fear. It will be clear at this stage that the small item clusters and sometimes unusual juxtapositions of items within factors in the Californian sample suggests strongly that there is great variation within the sample and few consistent dimensions of sexual attitudes.

Those dimensions that are consistent, however, are frequently common to both homosexual samples. Dimensions identifiable in both South Australian and Californian homosexual men include Libido and Control, Interest in Pornography, Comfort with Women, Permissiveness, Prudishness, and Fear of Sexual Relationships. Other dimensions that are sample-specific but that would appear to express important attitudinal dimensions, at least for the particular homosexual society in which they occur, are Lack of Monogamy (California) and Importance of Affect and Relationship (South Australia).

The generally dissimilar dimensions to those obtained in Eysenck's adult male sample suggest that sexual experience in homosexual men cannot be clustered in way similar to that of sexual experience in heterosexual men. The exceptions to this would appear to be the dimensions measuring Prudishness, Permissiveness, and Pornography. To a lessor degree, Sexual Excitement appears to be common to both homosexual and heterosexual men, but in differing forms. However, what is also clear is that in homosexual men these dimensions are truncated and contain many fewer items than the dimensions in heterosexuals. While dimensions appear to be more internally consistent in the South Australian homosexual men than in the Californian homosexual men, this may be function of the much greater diversity of homosexual attitudes and experiences in the San Francisco Bay area as compared with Adelaide, South Australia. Certainly, the small number of items in many of the dimensions obtained in homosexual men do not auger well for the reliability and stability of many of them, and it may be that attitudes toward sexuality in this group, as compared to heterosexual men, will be much more variable and to a large degree depend on the prevailing sociopolitical milieu in which the homosexual exists, as well as the nature and cohesiveness of the homosexual subcultures.

SEXUAL BEHAVIORS
AND SEXUAL ATTITUDES

The importance of sexual attitudes in psychovenereology is twofold: first, they are postulated to be dimensions underlying sexual behaviors that may increase risk of STD infection, and second, they may themselves be formed by social and psychological forces that are of interest. If sexual attitudes do underlie particular sexual behaviors that are associated with increased risk for STD infection, then they would be expected to be significantly different across these variables.

Investigation of the relationship between sexual attitudes and the three previously investigated sexual behaviors of partner numbers, sexual practices, and place of sexual contact reveals some consistent connections, which are revealed in Tables 9.3, 9.4, and 9.5. Table 9.3 illustrates the associations between the three categories of partner numbers per month (nil, one, and two or more) and the factor-scored sexual attitudes derived from the South Australian homosexual men. Six of the factors proved to be linked, with some of the relationships being in a nonlinear form.

TABLE 9.3 Relationship of Sexual Attitudes to Partner Numbers

Sexual Attitudes	Partner Numbers per month		
	0	1	2+
Factor 1: Fear of Sexual Relationships	19.8	18.2*	19.2
Factor 2: Interest in Pornography	9.2	10.3*	9.3
Factor 3: Sexual Excitement	8.2	9.1*	7.8
Factor 7: Prudishness	4.3	3.9*	4.3
Factor 8: Permissiveness	8.1	7.7	8.3*
Factor 9: Libido and Control	4.6	4.6	5.2*

*$p < .05$

Greater fear of sexual relationships was apparent in those with no partners and to a lesser extent those with multiple partners, suggesting that nil or multiple partners are both ways of coping with fear of sexual relationships, the former by not having any and the latter by having multiple and presumably emotionally shallow ones. Surprisingly, interest in pornography followed the same pattern, as did sexual excitement, which suggest strongly that those individuals who have a moderate number of sexual partners are those most sexually aroused. This would tend to suggest that multiple partner preference, at least within the context of these data, is not related only to sexual arousal, and that multiple partner number serve some other need. The significant difference between the multiple partner individuals and the other two groups on the scale measuring libido and control does suggest that those with multiple partners are less able to control sexual arousal when it does occur, possibly because other needs are activated that impart a more driven quality to the arousal. On the other hand, both those with nil and multiple partners are more prudish than those reporting a single partner on average per month, and those with multiple partners more permissive. These data, taken together, not only confirm that sexual attitudes are important associates (and presumably form an underlying dimension) of partner numbers, but also that both high and low partner numbers may be associated with having difficulty in relating to sexual partners. Those with least control of libido, not unexpectedly, have the highest numbers of partners.

Table 9.4 illustrates the relationship of sexual attitudes to specific sexual practices. It will be seen that three factors, Factor 2 (Interest in Pornography), Factor 8 (Permissiveness), and Factor 9 (Libido and Control) appear consistently across more than one sexual practice. A high frequency of oral sex appears to be associated with an increase in permissive attitudes and with an increase in interest in pornography. Permissiveness is also associated with an increased frequency of anal-insertor sex, along with an increased score on sexual excitement for those with high anal-insertor sex frequency. Anal intercourse-insertee is associated with an decreased score on libido and control (more control) and with a higher score on importance of affect and relationship, which strongly suggest that so-called passive anal intercourse is connected with better control and a greater importance placed on relational aspects of sexual encounters. Mutual masturbation also follows a different pattern altogether, with lower scores for interest in pornography and libido and control, suggesting

TABLE 9.4 Relationship of Sexual Attitudes to Sexual Practices

	High Frequency	Low Frequency
Oral Sex:		
Factor 2: Interest in Pornography	10.3	9.6+
Factor 8: Permissiveness	13.5	10.8*
Anal Intercourse-Insertor:		
Factor 3: Sexual Excitement	9.4	7.3**
Factor 8: Permissiveness	13.1	10.1**
Anal Intercourse-Insertee:		
Factor 6: Importance of Affect and Relationship	13.2	11.8*
Factor 9: Libido and Control	4.7	5.0*
Mutual Masturbation:		
Factor 2: Interest in Pornography	9.5	10.3*
Factor 9: Libido and Control	4.7	5.0+
Analingus:		
Factor 2: Interest in Pornography	10.2	9.5+
Factor 8: Permissiveness	8.3	7.9+

+p < .075
*p < .05
**p < .01

that such individuals are in better control of sexual impulses and less aroused by pornographic scenes or visual imagery. Those indulging in analingus, however, are both more aroused by pornographic scenes and, as might be expected, more permissive.

Permissiveness appears related to the exoticness of sexual activity and particularly to oral activity (fellatio and analingus), both of which are novel in the sense that oral-genital activity is often regarded as nonstandard by society. Mutual masturbation appears to occur in those with less arousal, and anal intercourse-insertee appears to be related with closer emotional liaisons. Again, it is clear that sexual attitudes are also linked to specific sexual practices, and in a way that appears to make some intuitive sense.

The relationship of sexual attitudes to places of partner contact appear in Table 9.5. Again, three factors, Factor 2 (Interest in Pornography), Factor 7 (Prudishness), and Factor 9 (Libido and Control), appear in more than one

TABLE 9.5 Relationship of Sexual Attitudes to Place of Partner Contact

	Contact	No Contact
Bars, Clubs, Discos:		
Factor 2: Interest in Pornography	10.4	9.5*
Factor 7: Prudishness	4.5	4.1+
Factor 9: Libido and Control	5.3	4.7**
Beats:		
Factor 5: Acceptance of Sexuality	8.3	7.2**
Factor 9: Libido and Control	4.3	4.8*
Work:		
Factor 2: Interest in Pornography	10.1	8.3**
Factor 7: Prudishness	4.3	3.9+
Factor 9: Libido and Control	5.0	4.3**
Friends:		
Factor 9: Libido and Control	4.6	4.9*
Sauna:		
Factor 6: Importance of Affect and Relationship	5.3	5.9+
Factor 8: Permissiveness	8.4	7.8*

+p < .075
*p < .05
**p < .01

category, and Factors 2 and 9 are also those appearing in the two previous analyses. Individuals attending bars, clubs, and discos for partner contact tend to have a greater interest in pornography and a higher score on Factor 9 indicating less control of libido. Those making sexual contacts cruising on beats appear to have better acceptance of their sexuality and better control of libido, while those making contact at work have greater interest in pornography, greater prudishness, and less control of libido. Individuals who meet partners through friends appear to have greater control of libido, while those who meet in saunas and bath houses are more permissive and place less importance on affect and relationships.

These data suggest that in the area of place of partner contact as well as in the other two areas already examined, sexual attitudes underlie sexual behaviors associated with degree of risk. What is of particular interest is that the same factors appear to underlie risk factors across sexual behaviors, namely, Libido and Control, and Interest in

Pornography. The presence of Libido and Control suggests strongly that the less controlled the individual's libido, the greater risk through sexual practices that transmit bodily fluids and the greater the risk of multiple partners. Factor 2, Interest in Pornography, in fact has the highest correlation with Factor 9 (-.43) and would appear to be tapping a similar dimension, which includes not only interest in pornography but also an emphasis on interest in sex and a degree of arousal by visual stimuli. While it is not particularly surprising that partner numbers, high-risk practices such as anal intercourse, and meeting partners at bars, clubs, and discos may be associated with this cluster of attitudes, it does clearly underscore the argument that understanding of sexual behaviors that place the individual at risk for STD infection will ultimately lie one step beyond the behaviors in the personality dimensions that underlie these and in the psychological and social forces that form attitudes and drive behaviors.

CONCLUSIONS

In conclusion, this chapter has illustrated not only that sexual attitudes in homosexual men differ in terms of structure and meaning from those in heterosexual men, but also that there is a wide degree of variation within homosexual men. While the dimensions obtained were more consistent in the South Australian sample, there are clearly major dimensions underlying sexual attitudes in homosexual men regardless of context. These common dimensions include Interest in Pornography and in sex, implying a visual arousal factor, degree of Libido and Control, attitudes toward relationships in terms of both affect and exclusiveness, and the more general dimensions of prudishness and permissiveness found also in heterosexual males.

Looking at all three areas of sexual behavior which are thought to mediate risk of STD infection (partner numbers, sexual practices, and places of sexual contact), many of these dimensions significantly differentiated groups. Of particular discriminating power were the related dimensions of Libido and Control and Interest in Pornography (which also includes interest in sex). Clearly, sexual attitudes are intimately associated with, and probably underlie, risk-related sexual behaviors, and future research in the area of psychovenereology will undoubtedly begin to concentrate on these personality-related variables in an attempt to understand the determinants of sexual behavior as they relate to STDs.

10

The Multiple Meanings of
Sexually Related Disease Infections

There have been many assumptions made about STDs and
their social and societal bases, and it is unfortunate that
many of the beliefs about venereal diseases continue to be
the unquestioned basis of many research hypotheses. Nor
has it been sufficiently recognized that psychological
concommitants and sequelae of STD infection are based
solidly on the social and individual perception of the meaning of STDs.

It has been recognized for some time that the meaning
of any disease to the individual is one of the most important
determinants of the subsequent illness behaviors, reactions
to illness, attribution of responsibility for the illness, and
compliance with treatment. Groddeck (1929) has argued
that the *meaning* of the illness to the individual is one of
central importance in understanding the individual's reaction
to it. He suggests that flight into illness (as opposed to
contracting an infection) has a number of advantages,
including repression of conflicts and as a means of punishing oneself for perceived sins. Groddeck also points out
that illness, both in terms of its presence and its form, is
a useful expression of the individual's psychology. Given
that the meaning of the illness determines the individual's
response to it and future avoidance and risk-related behaviors, it is central to the understanding of STDs in homosexual men to understand the meaning of contracting STDs
in this population. Venereal disease has always had very
specific and well-known connotations from biblical times on:

171

Rosebury (1972) argues strongly that the leprosy of the Old and New Testaments was actually syphilis from its descriptions in the Bible and in subsequent reports to 1494. Rosebury also points out that sex has generally been considered dirty, and venereal disease dirty in its own right; he concludes that the combination is almost untouchable. Add to this untouchable combination a form of sexual expression (homosexuality) which has until recently been considered a perversion and made illegal in many jurisdictions as well as condemned in most religious movements, and the mixture is guaranteed to have a severe and negative influence.

Rosebury cogently reviews the notion of venereal diseases as first an indication of God's punishment through to the present description of STDs as a "disease of society," a description that has strong moral overtones. He notes as historical examples that Henry VIII of England and Casanova were believed to have "deserved" to have venereal disease as a punishment for their sins, but that this argument was not used for Keats or Schubert, who also contracted venereal disease (but who apparently were exceptions if individuals "deserved" STDs as a punishment for sin!). So pervasive was the belief that venereal diseases were punishment that Rosebury notes that the production of Ibsen's *Ghosts* in London in the 1880s shocked audiences because it portrayed diseases and death, not as the wages of sin, but as punishment for virtue! As a parallel to this, Rosebury also notes adolescents were warned not only that masturbation was sinful, but that it was physically harmful as well. The works of most late nineteenth century neurologists and sexologists such as von Krafft-Ebing (1886/1965) are full of descriptions of mental illness that resulted from masturbation. This, Rosebury notes, is not far removed from the argument of Astruc in the mid-eighteenth century that venereal disease was a "punishment for the lewdness of mankind." The satirist Samuel Butler (1872/1935) described a society in which crime was considered an illness, and illness a crime. In illustrating the absurdities of the Victorian legal and medical systems, however, he came close to describing attitudes to venereal diseases, in which contracting an illness was indeed considered a crime.

Modern venereology, argues Rosebury, is no different, with one medical practitioner suggesting in 1955 that long and disagreeable treatments which were no longer necessary with the advent of penicillin were preferable in that they punished promiscuity, and another practioner in 1963 referring to gonococci as "God's little helpers." Perhaps the best description of medical attitudes to STDs in the recent past is a graphic description by Burns in his 1947 work *The Gallery*, cited by Rosebury, which portrays the attitude of an army doctor in World War II to venereal disease treatment:

> I don't say: welcome to our hospital. You're not going to have a good time here. Our whole setup is guaranteed to make you hate everything about us. We don't want men coming back here, do you see? There's no excuse for getting VD. No excuse whatever. We give you treatment here, but we do it in such a way that you won't care to come back as a repeater. . . .

Rosebury, however, notes that from the advent of penicillin, venereologists were learning to think of syphilis scientifically as a dangerous communicable disease rather than moralistically as a punishment for sin. Nevertheless, Nicol (1963) was able to suggest in the prestigious *British Journal of Venereal Diseases* that perhaps we should "accept that God has provided these disincentives (VD) to promiscuity . . . Should we, as mere mortals, remove them?" It is clear that much of this attitude remains in the mind of the general public, and has been resurrected with the advent of AIDS in numerous pronouncements, with some deluded clerics going so far as to suggest that God has sent AIDS to punish wanton sexual behavior since man had rendered syphilis treatable. In contrast, Pankhurst (1913) argued, in the context of the female suffragette, that venereal disease arose from male institutions such as prostitution and promiscuity, and that the cure for venereal disease was "votes for women and chastity for men." However, more in line with social and religious attitudes to STDs at the time, she also argues that nature had "decreed a punishment for sexual immorality such as she imposes in respect of no other sin."

Venereologists, however, had moved from the belief that STDs were a punishment for sexual behavior to the concept of social diseases, which removed God but retained the moral indignation. Social diseases existed where sexual contact led to physical harm, and Rosebury in fact notes that the treponematoses probably actually developed out of human social *progress,* and particularly from the habit of communal living and close social interaction. He suggests that this emphasis on social issues rather than health still focused on the repression and punishment of the individual rather than on the pathogen, but the transgression was social rather than religious. Unfortunately, this has led to general medical practitioners not reporting STDs in an attempt to protect patients from what is considered a "crime" by society, since their patients do not fit the stereotype of "social criminals." Other scientists have suggested that society in general, by refraining from moral sanctions, has smoothed the sexual path that is made more attractive by films, the press, dress, and cosmetic firms. The remedy, it is suggested, is no premarital or extra-marital intercourse.

At this point, the idea of STD victims being pre-disposed to venereal infection becomes more important, since a social disease requires socially related causes. At the individual level, Morton (1966), in his discussion of venereal diseases as a social problem, suggests that lack of an intelligent and affectionate approach by parents is a predisposing factor, and goes on to state that for every girl impelled to promiscuity by these external factors, a girl in precisely similar circumstances can be found who has resisted them, individual character and psychological make-up being the final determining factor. Thus, venereal disease is linked with patterns of inappropriate social development, including parental rearing patterns and ex-ternal pressures from the forces of big business and the cinema.

The third step in medical thinking on the genesis of STD infection is to remove the moral disintegration from the individual to the society at large. Rosebury cites a World Health Organization document of 1968 which links the in-crease in STDs to increasing social change, including technological development, war, industrialization, and urbanization. The implication is that social change promotes stress and insecurity, which in turn may be mitigated by sexual contacts. The World Health Organization document also makes it clear that there is a second route for the increase in STDs implicated, which is the coexisting eco-nomic, social, and sexual emancipation that makes sex more available and less stigmatized. The root of the social problem, Rosebury suggests, is to be found as much in the older generation as in the young. He argues that re-pression persists as a vestige of puritanism, while stimu-lation of sexual appetites operates by the display of sex and by its exploitation for profit. Persistence of a double standard itself adds stresses, particularly if venereal disease is seen as "bad" and sexual expression as accept-able. The major issue that Rosebury (1972) identified in STD control was that morals should be emphasized more than microbes (by "morals" he refers to habits of life or modes of conduct). He goes on to note that epidemiolog-ically, there appear to be no national differences in terms of those societies that report STD incidence, which sug-gests that societal influences cannot be blamed for STD infections to any great extent.

There is perhaps a fourth stage to be considered after the blaming of social forces that lead to at-risk behavior: the belief that STDs should be treated just as any other infectious disease. It is interesting that Rosebury argues that the treponematoses developed along with ubanization, since it could be argued that STDs are a social disease along with influenza, rubella, the common cold, and many other infectious diseases that are not associated with stigma pertaining to their origin. The STDs are stigmatized solely with regard to their origin in sexual behavior, and in circumstances where it is clear that they were not sexually contracted; for example, by careless medical or laboratory practices such as needle sticks or by close contact such as parent-child interactions there is less stigma attached. Why, then, should STDs not be seen as a risk of human social and physical behavior in the same way as rubella, infectious mononucleosis, chicken pox, and other infections associated with human contact of varying degrees of phys-ical proximity? Why should we spend time attempting to explain at-risk behavior for STDs and not, for example, looking at demographic, psychological correlates of individu-als who have contracted influenza? These arguments are raised by individuals to whom STDs are a fact of life and treated, in some cases, with greater ease than the common cold. Other individuals will react with disbelief on con-tracting an STD, since they believe that such infection is shameful and occurs only in the promiscuous. Since their self-definition is not one of promiscuity, they may then see the STD as just another infection because they do not fit the common stereotype. Other individuals may change their self-definition, usually if they have tended to see STDs as a punishment for sin. Possibly the strongest influence on patient reaction is the reaction of the treating medical practitioner. For this reason, it is important to look at some of the philosophies of medicine that may determine medical attitudes to STDs.

In a review of the scientific and medical developments that led to the Wasserman test, Fleck (1935/1979) argues that concepts are not spontaneously created but are de-termined by their "ancestors," for instance, the concepts that preceded them. In the case of STDs, Fleck suggests that our scientific knowledge is culturally conditioned, and that collective thought patterns form around organized social groups. If these groups are sufficiently large and exist long enough, the thought style becomes fixed and formal, and is accepted as a scientific fact. In the case of venereal diseases, Fleck argues, the old beliefs that STDs were a punishment for sin was translated into medical thought and STDs regarded as a particular disease entity and not just as the result of particular pathogens (although the appropriate pathogen was a necessary cause). This development of a concentration on the venereal and sinful aspects of venereal disease has thus led to consideration of cofactors as equally important as the causative organism. Fleck contrasts venereal disease in this regard with tuberculosis, which was seen as a "romantic" disease, and notes the consequent paucity of the research on tuberculosis with the extensive research on venereal disease, particularly syphilis, which culminated in the development both of the Wasserman test and the discovery of Salvarsan. Fleck also points out that observation without assumptions is nonsense in the context of most scientific thought, and illustrates this in the case of syphilis, where he describes how fixed and restrictive notions of "bad blood" lead to fixed areas of investigation, in this case the discovery of the Wasserman blood test. However, Fleck's argument is also equally applicable to modern research into STDs. We have preserved the medical model that was formerly based on sin for STDs in much the same way that we have translated homosexuality from sin to mental illness. Thus we tend to look at STDs, and particularly their behavioral and psychological concommitants, as if they were still a punishment for religious or social deviance. In doing this, we are falling into what Burns (1974) calls an ontological fallacy: we are transmuting intellectual constructs that had their roots in prescientific religious thought into perceptual realities (much as the humors of ancient Greek medicine became realities for the medieval physician).

Kuhn (1972) has used arguments similar to those of Fleck (1935/1979), suggesting that we tend to test within models rather than between them. It could certainly be argued that in looking at the psychological and social contexts of STD infection we are still testing within the old sin and deviance model of STDs that has been medicalized, and that there is no necessary reason why we should expect to find more deviant or abnormal social backgrounds or psychological variables in STD-infected individuals than in, say, those with one or more episodes of upper respiratory tract infections (leaving aside, for the moment, psychosomatic illness and interactions between psychological variables and immune status). However, we should also recognize, as Comaroff (1982) has pointed out, that looking at the dichotomy of person and context reduces environmental variables in multifactorial models of disease, and therefore reduces responsibility for illness from contradictions in the sociocultural domain to conflicts within the person. Comaroff argues that such a dichotomy between person and context fosters the rationale that the sick and the disadvantaged suffer as a result of biological inadequacy or their own psychological inadequacy.

With the recognition that there are many assumptions about STDs which we accept as scientific fact without querying either their origin or whether they are essential to the hypotheses we are adopting, we are able to recognize alternative models to test between. In discussing the meaning of STDs to the individual, we have identified at least four separate models.

1. STDs are a deserved outcome of indiscriminate sexual behavior and punishment for sexual sins.
2. STDs are a consequence of individual inadequacy that leads to sexually indiscriminate behavior.
3. STDs are a consequence of a breakdown in traditional social values and rapid social change.
4. STDs are the result of an individual coming into intimate contact with a virulent pathogen.

Note that there is a heirarchy of blame from model 1 to model 4. The heirarchy of blame is a concommitant of a similar heirarchy of the degree to which the individual is responsible for the infection. It is almost impossible to investigate social and psychological associations with STD infection and not have an implicit model underlying one's hypotheses. One must also recognize that different models will apply in different cultures, and will depend on the degree to which sexual behavior is cathected (that is, the degree to which there is a psychological investment in it).

More important, the meaning of STDs to the patient and to a lesser degree the attending health professional will affect not only the compliance with treatment, but also the psychological sequelae and the subsequent risks of exposure to STDs the individual takes. These may be examined by reference to the four models proposed.

STD AS PUNISHMENT

When the individual sees the STD as punishment, there is a good chance that they have had a particularly religious background or have never come to terms with sexuality. In the case of the homosexual man, the individual will probably be at one of the first three stages of homosexual adjustment described by Cass (1979), in which their sexual orientation is not usually publicly acknowledged and almost invariably not accepted. The combination of the stigma of STD along with the stigma of homosexuality is an extremely powerful one, and the homosexual STD patient who sees his infection as an indication that he is being punished will need careful attention. The result of infection is likely to include remorse or sometimes clinical or subclinical depression as the individual is faced with the evidence of a sexual behavior that he has probably compartmentalized or denied. In such cases the anxiety or embarrassment may lead to defaulting from treatment, or denial of a homosexual orientation in the first place. Ross (1985b) has noted that some 20 percent of STD clinic attenders who are homosexual deny their real sexual orientation to the attending physician, and that these individuals are most likely to expect the most negative reactions to their sexuality from others. Such individuals are also most likely to be first attenders, and where they also attend private physicians rather than public clinics, may tend to deny their sexuality to a greater extent. It is important that the attending physician does not accept or reinforce the patient's negative view of his sexuality, particularly as this may be one of the first times the patient has admitted his sexual orientation to anyone outside of a small circle. Other cases where the patient has apparently accepted his sexuality may occur with some of the more severe STDs: as an example, some AIDS sufferers who have been living openly homosexual lives have seen their disease as a "punishment from God" and blamed it on their homosexuality. The combination of homosexuality and STDs is a powerful one, and for the patient's mental well-being, if it is apparent that they see their STD infection as a "punishment," some attempt at reassurance and correction must be made. In some severe cases, it is helpful to have access to accepting clergy for referral.

This first category of the meaning of infection to the individual is most notable for its mental health consequences, which in many cases require more attention than the STD. Venereophobia, in which there is no evidence of STD infection but the patient is convinced that infection has occurred, most commonly occurs in patients who see it as punishment for some real or imagined misdeed, usually of a sexual nature.

STD AS EVIDENCE OF MALADJUSTMENT

This second category has much in common with the first category in which STDs are seen as a punishment. While the reason for the individual's dysphoria on realizing that he has an STD is a result of lack of acceptance of his sexual orientation, the basis is not religious and the dysphoria not so pronounced. Nevertheless, the major sequelae of note are also likely to be in mental status, but denial through compartmentalization of sexual orientation may also be present. Married men frequently fall into this category, and their homosexual activities are thus likely to occur in public toilets (Humphreys in 1970 found that 54 percent of men who had sex in public toilets were married). As a result, the contacts are often likely to be unknown, and there is the added complication that the patient's wife may have been infected, and be unaware of her spouse's bisexuality. Since a sizeable proportion of homosexual men (between 10 and 20 percent) marry, and since those who marry are usually those less accepting of their homosexuality (Ross 1978, 1983), such individuals may be frequently represented in those with sexual orientation dysphorias. In contrast to ego-dystonic homosexuality (where individuals are unhappy at being homosexual), however, such patients become disturbed by their sexuality only when it produces negative consequences such as STD infection.

A second group within this category are those with mild dysphoria on infection, and who recognize that there is nothing they can do about their sexual orientation but feel that it might be easier to be heterosexual. They rarely present a problem in terms of either compliance with treatment or mental state. On the other hand, too great a degree of dysphoria may result in sexual contacts that are anonymous since having known partners and affective contact could be too guilt engendering. Contact tracing is thus likely to be difficult, although returning for proof of cure is usually not a problem.

STDs AS THE FAULT OF A SICK SOCIETY

In this group, the blame for STD infection is likely to be projected rather than introjected, and the individual is most likely to be at Cass's (1979) fifth stage of homosexual development. The fifth stage, according to Cass, is the period where the individual accepts his homosexuality and defines his whole lifestyle in terms of it. Thus, to the extent where he allocates blame for STD infection, it cannot lie with his sexual orientation, which is so centrally important to him, but must lie elsewhere. Elsewhere is usually the society that so stigmatizes homosexuals that they are forced to meet in secluded places and have impersonal sexual contacts. Stigmatization may also affect the number of sexual partners by lowering self-esteem to the point where relationships are not possible, and multiple partners help to assuage a negative self-image. While these arguments are based on reality in countries where homosexuality is severly stigmatized and legal penalties are severe, they seldom apply to those whose homosexuality is the central defining construct of their lifestyle. Essentially, those who believe that STDs are the fault of a discriminatory society are unable to accept that any fault lies with them, and are thus unresponsive to suggestions about cutting down at-risk practices. In some cases, such a suggestion will be construed as a condemnation of their homosexuality, and the medical interaction terminated. In others, STD infection becomes a red badge of courage, indicating emancipation from the restrictive and bourgeois sexual habits of monogamy and possession of sexual partners. Where sexual behavior is seen as a political or social statement, it is most unlikely that it will be open to modification.

Similarly, where an individual has "come out" recently as a homosexual, it is most likely that there will be more frequent sexual contacts both in response to a previous deficit of sexual contact in most cases, and because the predominant understanding of homosexuality centers on its sexual component rather than its affective or social component. In such cases, sexual activity may be higher than it would otherwise be due to an affirmation of the individual's core identity. If this is the case, then suggestions that attempt to modify sexual behavior could be seen as a rejection of their homosexuality, and thus the point should be cautiously broached. Usually individuals move on to Cass's stage 6, and the issue is not so fraught with danger. If, however, this does not appear to be occurring after a lapse of several years, it may be advisable to raise the issue by ascertaining the meaning of sexual behavior to the patient and by attempting to identify any personal difficulties that may be driving their sexual behavior. Generally, this stage is the opposite of the STD as Punishment group, in that the latter see their sexuality as inviting retribution while the former see their sexuality as a central and positive aspect of their lifestyle.

STDs AS JUST ANOTHER INFECTION

For some individuals, STD infection is not highly cathected and carries no investment in psychic energy. Such individuals are likely to be in Cass's stage 5 or stage 6, in which a homosexual orientation is seen as being only one of many identifications the individual has, and not central to identity or lifestyle. Of course, STD infection medically *is* just another infection with varying risks associated, but few people are able to see it that way. In terms of dealing with individuals at this stage of STD perception, there is little problem in making suggestions of modification of at-risk behaviors, but on the other hand if infection is not cathected, there is little reason to do so unless the risk is a major one (such as with hepatitis B or AIDS).

People who fall into this category tend to have identified themselves as homosexual for longer and to approach sexuality in a fairly hedonistic way. Thus, if modification to partner numbers as a response to AIDS is necessary, partner numbers may be cut down without great psychological trauma. However, if partner numbers are important to the person to maintain self-esteem, then that individual probably falls into the category of seeing STDs as the "fault of a sick society."

While the aim of venerologists should be to remove the psychological involvement to the point where STDs are just another infectious disease, the attendant consequence is to also remove the pressures, positive and negative, on individuals to modify their behaviors. Pressure to modify behavior will thus be a consequence of the risks that STDs carry (for example, high risk for AIDS, low for gonorrhea). However, by now it will have been recognized that patients are not the only ones with beliefs about STDs.

MEDICAL REACTIONS TO STDs

Each of the four stages described can also be used to describe medical attitudes to STD infection. Those who have read widely on the subject will be able to classify various authors and authorities on a continuum from seeing the gonococcus as "God's little helpers" through to approaching it as just a part of infectious disease management. The important thing to note is that our attitudes as health-care professionals will affect not only our approach to our patients but, as pointed out in Chapter 4, our own attitudes will interact with those of our patients. Thus, the best physician-patient interaction will result from the closest positions on the continuum, while the most hostile and clinically inappropriate ones will result from the widest separation of beliefs about the meaning of STDs of the patient and the physician.

The major thrust of this chapter has been to identify the scientific trends that occur with regard to views on STDs, to point out that our hypotheses are not value-free, and to show that our assumptions about what are scientific "facts" will determine both the context and the findings of our research. At a clinical level, it is a mistake of equal magnitude to assume that there are not multiple meanings attached to STDs, both on the part of our patients and, hopefully to a lesser extent, on the part of the physician. Appropriate patient management requires that the psychological and social context of the illness be considered, and given the heavily cathected nature of sexuality, and the even more heavily cathected nature of homosexuality, it could be argued that the psychological aspect of management is of equal importance as the medical side. Certainly the attitude of the attending physician will have an important role in the decision of the patient to reattend, and to his own attitude to alteration of at-risk behaviors (if appropriate) and to STDs. Ultimately, we must recognize that if the meaning of the illness is central to the individual's response to it and thus to his subsequent health-related behaviors, then STDs must rank with the life-threatening illnesses in terms of the emotions engendered and the defenses activated in a large number of homosexual men if not in the majority of people.

11

Illness Behavior in Sexually Transmitted Disease Infections

Illness behavior, or lack of it, in attenders at sexually transmitted disease clinics has important implications for both diagnosis and treatment. In the case of individuals with an erroneous conviction that they have a sexually transmitted disease, which Hart (1977) refers to as venereoneurosis, there is abnormal illness behavior in terms of both general hypochondriasis and a strong disease conviction without any demonstrable pathology, as well as an indication that the patient feels responsible for, or deserves, an illness (Bhanji and Mahony 1978). In the case of other individuals, and perhaps more common, is the refusal to see a sexually transmitted disease as an illness but rather as a nuisance or a minor nonsignificant risk of a particular lifestyle. Clinical observation has tended to suggest that in the case of the absence of illness behavior, patients will frequently compromise treatment by discontinuing medication after symptoms have resolved, continuing sexual activity after symptom resolution but before a clearance, or not returning for proof of cure. Thus, both abnormal illness behavior and lack of illness behavior may have implications for treatment and management of individuals with sexually transmitted diseases.

For these reasons, examination of abnormal illness behavior in attenders at sexually transmitted disease clinics is important. Not only do we need to know whether illness behaviors as we know them in other diseases exist in STDs, but if they do exist, what is abnormal? Are there any differences between homosexuals and heterosexuals in this regard?

The concept of illness behavior has been developed by Pilowsky (1969, 1978). Illness behavior is generally defined as the ways in which symptoms may be differentially perceived, evaluated, and acted (or not acted) on by different kinds of persons. This includes inappropriate or maladaptive modes of response to one's state of health, such as (in the classic situations) hypochondriasis and symptom preoccupation, neurasthenia, and conversion reactions. In patients with STDs, particularly with venereoneurotics, this abnormal illness behavior makes treatment difficult, and it is important not to reinforce the symptoms by repeated testing for pathogens and other medical interventions. Instead, it is necessary to concentrate on the psychological state that underlies the venereoneurosis: this is usually one of two factors. First, there is guilt about a particular sexual activity (or class of activities, such as homosexuality) and STD infection is seen as a deserved punishment. Second, there may be a disease phobia that manifests itself in obsessive checking of the genitals and attention to the most minute changes in bodily function. This is equivalent to hypochondriasis focused on other anatomical sites, and is often sufficiently obsessional and frequent as to cause urethral inflammation and discharge (Hart 1977).

Abnormal illness behavior, however, can also occur at the opposite end of the spectrum, with an underreaction to illness. The classic example is "la belle indifférence" in cases of conversion reaction, in which the individual appears unconcerned by a disabling lack of function of a limb or limbs or organ system. In the case of STD infections, this abnormal underreaction often manifests itself with total lack of concern over the disease acquired, and similar lack of concern over attending for proof of cure, continuing courses of treatment, or infection of subsequent partners. In the case of STD infection, however, this is usually denial rather than indifference. However, in order to be able to classify abnormal illness behavior in STD clinic attenders, and particularly homosexual men, it is necessary first to assess the range of *normal* illness behavior in STD clinic attenders. This is best achieved using the Illness Behavior Questionnaire of Pilowsky and Spence (1983).

The Illness Behavior Questionnaire is a 62-item inventory consisting of one- or two-line questions dealing with health-related attitudes, perceptions and behaviors and requiring a yes/no response to be circled. Examples of selected questions appear in Table 11.1. Pilowsky developed the Illness Behavior Questionnaire to measure

TABLE 11.1   Items Left Blank Most Frequently in the Illness Behavior
Questionnaire

Item Number	Number Cases Left Blank	Question
13	25	If you feel ill or worried, can you be cheered up by the doctor?
23	26	Do people feel sorry for you when you are ill?
32	26	Are you upset by the way people take your illness?
39	25	Do you get the feeling people are not taking your illness seriously enough?
44	25	Do you think there is something the matter with your mind?
50	24	Do you often have the symptoms of a serious disease?
53	25	Do you prefer to keep your feelings to yourself?
55	26	Would all your worries be over if you were physically healthy?
56	26	Are you more irritable toward other people?
57	25	Do you think that your symptoms may be caused by worry?

seven subsets of illness behavior: General Hypochondriasis
(phobic concern about state of health), Disease Conviction
(affirmation that physical disease exists and symptom preoccupation), Psychological versus Somatic Perception of
Illness (belief in the presence of a psychological component
of the illness for high scorers), Affective Inhibition (difficulty in expressing personal feelings), Affective Disturbance (feelings of anxiety or sadness), Denial (of life
stresses and blaming all problems on the illness), and
Irritability (presence of angry feelings and interpersonal
friction). Scores on subscales of the Illness Behavior
Questionnaire can be used to measure individual differences
in illness behavior (Pilowsky and Spence 1983) and to
compare patient groups with other known patient groups.
    In the investigation described in this chapter, it was
hypothesized that there would be less illness behavior
(particularly General Hypochondriasis and Psychological
versus Somatic Perception of Illness) in those individuals

who had previously had a sexually transmitted disease.
This would be a result of being desensitized to the impact
of STD infections. Second, it was hypothesized that illness
behavior would be lower in individuals with higher partner
numbers; such individuals would tend to regard STD infection as an unimportant risk and one worth taking.
Third, it was hypothesized that illness behavior would be
higher in those individuals who attended with symptoms
compared with check-up attenders, since such people would
have an actual illness. Finally, it was hypothesized that
homosexual men would show less illness behavior since they
would be more aware of STDs and probably exposed to them
more frequently, and because it appeared that STDs were
more commonly discussed in homosexual publications.

METHOD

Questionnaires were handed to all daytime attenders over a
one-week period in July (midwinter) at a public sexually
transmitted disease clinic in Adelaide, South Australia, a
city of 1 million inhabitants. The clinic was the central one
of three city clinics, and located opposite a major university
hospital. It was, however, distant from residential areas.
The questionnaire was headed, "Survey of Health Attitudes
in Sexually Transmissible Disease Clinics," and instructions
were:

> We are carrying out some work on the attitudes and
> feelings of people attending Sexually Transmissible
> Disease Clinics in Adelaide, in an attempt to find
> out more about our patients and their needs. We
> would be grateful if you would quickly fill out the
> enclosed questionnaire: it is anonymous and we do
> not want you to put your name on it. Please hand
> it to the doctor or nurse when you go in. We
> thank you in advance for your co-operation.

Details requested included age, sex, partner preference as
measured by the Kinsey Scale (Kinsey, Pomeroy and Martin
1948), number of partners in the preceding month, reason
for attendance, occupation, and number of previous episodes of a sexually transmitted disease. The form was then
handed to the attending medical officer who noted number
and nature of previous diagnoses and present diagnosis.
Since a pilot study had revealed that many attenders gave
the demographic data outlined above but refused to complete
the Illness Behavior Questionnaire, stating that it was not

appropriate to them as they were not ill, noncompletion or partial completion of the Illness Behavior Questionnaire was included as a variable measuring another aspect of illness behavior, namely, a refusal to see oneself as ill.

SAMPLE

The sample consisted of 90 males and 47 females, mean ages 27.14±7.39, range 17–53 (males) and 27.9±9.12, range 15–54 (females). Reasons for attendance were routine checkup, 20.7 percent; symptoms of VD, 21.5 percent; contact, 7.4 percent; concern that they might have VD, 39.3 percent; and other (for example, a medical illness) 11.1 percent. Occupational cases were professional and managerial, 30.6 percent; clerical scales 10.4 percent; skilled trade, 16.4 percent; unskilled worker, 9 percent; unemployed, 17.9 percent; home duties, 5.2 percent; prostitute, 4.5 percent; and student, 6 percent. Number of sexual partners in the past month ranged from 0 to 300: excluding the responses of the prostitutes (10–300), the median was 1.53. Range of number of times patients reported a previous sexually transmitted disease was 0–20 (median 0.92), and number of previous diagnoses in the case notes ranged from 0–14 (median 1.04). Current diagnoses were gonorrhea, 2.5 percent; nongonococcal urethritis, 19.8 percent; genital warts, 9.0 percent; herpes, 4.1 percent; dermatological disorder, 4.1 percent; candida, trichomonas, 12.3 percent; anxiety, 3.3 percent; and checkup only without diagnosis, 46.3 percent.

Data analysis consisted of computing Pearson product-moment correlation coefficients between the eight Illness Behavior Questionnaire subscales plus the Conscious Exaggeration subscale (Clayer, Bookless and Ross 1984) and age, partner numbers in previous month (excluding prostitutes), number of previous times respondents had had a sexually transmitted disease, and number of previous diagnoses at the clinic (taken from the clinic notes). An index of degree of completion of the questionnaire was also computed as a percentage. t tests were computed between the groups of those with and without a current diagnosis, those who had had a sexually transmitted disease previously and those who had not, those with nil or one partner in the previous month and those with more than one, and the Illness Behavior Questionnaire subscales. Demographic variables (age, partner numbers, previous infections, case note records of previous diagnoses) were also compared on t test between those who had completed more than 93 percent of the questionnaire and those who had completed less than this (an arbitrary figure derived from the fact that one-third had not answered five or more questions).

RESULTS

Data revealed that 29.2 percent of the respondents had completed 92 percent or less of the questionnaire, and those items that were left blank at more than one standard deviation above the mean frequency of nonresponding (18.23±5.60) appear in Table 11.1. Means and standard deviations of the Illness Behavior Questionnaire subscales appear in Table 11.2, and Table 11.3 illustrates the differences between the groups with previous sexually transmitted diseases, high versus low partner numbers in the past month, and previous versus no previous diagnoses at the clinic. Correlations between the Illness Behavior Questionnaire scales and demographic variables were all insignificant with the exceptions of psychological versus somatic perceptions of illness (.18), the Whiteley Index of Hypochondriasis (.19), Irritability (-.19), and previous number of clinic diagnoses (all $p < .05$). There were no significant differences on t test between those who had had a diagnosis made at the clinic on the visit at which they filled out the questionnaire and those with no abnormalities detected on the Illness Behavior Subscales subscales or previous episodes of STDs, number of diagnoses made previously at the clinic, or number of partners in the past month. Those who completed more than 93 percent of the questionnaire were more likely to report more previous STD episodes (1.11±2.66 vs 0.42±0.68, $t = 2.38$, $p < .05$). Comparison between homosexual and heterosexual patients (Table 11.4 and 11.5) revealed that there were differences on three scales of the Illness Behavior Questionnaire, Affective Inhibition, Depression, and the Whitely Index of Hypochondriasis.

DISCUSSION

From these data, it can be seen that the results are in fact contrary to the hypotheses. Table 11.3 illustrates clearly that those individuals who have reported the most previous episodes of a sexually transmitted disease are likely to score *higher* on General Hypochondriasis and thus display a higher level of arousal and anxiety about their illness or clinic attendance. It may be that previous episodes have

TABLE 11.2   Illness Behavior Questionnaire Subscales (Mean ± SDs)

	Males	Females
General Hypochondriasis	2.82±2.14*	2.92±1.52*
Disease Conviction	1.89±1.24	1.77±1.15
Psychological vs Somatic Perception	2.13±0.79	2.15±0.80
Affective Inhibition	2.84±1.21*	2.52±1.39
Affective Disturbance	2.55±1.49*	2.81±1.38
Denial	2.95±1.41	2.89±1.37+
Irritability	2.32±1.46	2.24±1.13
Whiteley Index of Hypochondriasis	4.48±3.17	4.00±2.82*
Conscious Exaggeration	5.61±4.38	5.84±3.19

*Significantly higher than Adelaide general practice patients (p < .05).
+Significantly lower than Adelaide general practice patients (p < .05).

sensitized such individuals to changes in body function. It is also particularly noteworthy that presence as opposed to absence of a diagnosed sexually transmitted disease did not produce any significant difference in any of the Illness Behavior Questionnaire subscales. Those with higher previous numbers of infections also tended to deny life stresses more, and attribute their problems to the illness, as well as to display significantly higher disease conviction (including symptom preoccupation), affective disturbance (anxiety and sadness), and higher levels of exaggeration of their symptoms.

In addition, as might be expected, they tended to be older and to have had more clinic diagnoses of sexually transmitted disease. This last point suggests that the individual's assessment of the number of previous STD infections is accurate since it is significantly related to the number of diagnoses of sexually transmitted diseases noted in the clinic records. It is thus clear that those with a history of previous episodes of a sexually transmitted disease are *more* likely to display illness behavior than new cases.

A tentative explanation for this may be found in Table 11.3 by examining the Illness Behavior Questionnaire subscales differentiating those with the greatest number of partners in the past month. Such individuals tend to score higher on the scale Psychological versus Somatic Perception of Illness measuring the degree of the patient's recognizing a psychological component of (and perhaps feeling they

TABLE 11.3 Significant Differences Between Groups on Illness Behavior
Questionnaire Subscales and Previous History

Partner Numbers in Past Month:	< 2	> 2
Psychological vs Somatic Perception	2.32±0.74	2.02±0.80*
Denial	2.59±1.37	3.14±1.37*
Whiteley Index of Hypochondriasis	5.00±3.09	3.84±2.93*
Times Previous VD	1.44±3.40	0.57±0.97*
Previous Clinic Diagnoses	2.90±2.83	1.45±0.80**
Previous Venereal Disease Episodes:	< 1	0
General Hypochondriasis	4.08±2.31	2.60±1.75*
Disease Conviction	2.28±1.23	1.73±1.18*
Affective Disturbance	2.97±1.50	2.86±1.31*
Conscious Exaggeration	7.67±4.85	5.20±3.59*
Age	29.74±7.78	25.87±7.82**
Previous Clinic Diagnoses	2.33±2.30	1.31±0.79
Previous Clinic Diagnoses:	< 2	> 2
Age	29.69±7.47	26.79±8.07*
Times Previous Venereal Disease	2.97±4.19	0.34±0.66**

*p < .05
**p < .01

deserve) the illness, as well as denying life stresses. Such individuals are probably guilty about the possibility of having contracted a sexually transmitted disease, thus are anxious to attribute their problems to this rather than to other life stresses. As a consequence, rather than the isolated episode of sexually transmitted disease inducing illness behavior, it would appear that the more episodes of disease, the greater the subsequent illness behavior. These data tend to suggest that some aspects of illness behavior are an additive response to previous illness, which is confirmed by the modest but significant correlations between previous number of diagnoses and both psychological perceptions of the illness and the Whiteley Index of Hypochondriasis. These data also suggest that the meaning of the illness may change as it is seen as being less a chance event (which are probably seen as somatic concerns) and more due to factors within the individual's control, given that it has reoccurred.

Seen in this context, the finding that those who declined to complete the Illness Behavior Questionnaire are more likely to be first attenders does suggest that noncompletion should be seen as a denial of presence of illness-related behavior or denial of the fact that a sexually transmitted disease is an illness. From a clinical point of view, then, these data suggest that those at greatest risk of failing to comply with a treatment regime or to reattend for proof of cure are likely to be first attenders rather than persistent attenders: efforts should thus be concentrated on first attenders to ensure compliance. It may also be the case that denial of illness is tantamount to denial of the fact of having contracted a sexually transmitted disease, and may be associated with the trauma of the discovery that one has a socially unacceptable disorder.

The socially unacceptable nature of sexually related infections is well illustrated in Table 11.1, in that those ten questions most commonly left blank refer to the public aspect of the illness. It is apparent that individuals feel that questions about reactions to an illness that is probably not discussed with anybody, as well as suggestions that the infection is psychologically determined, are inappropriate. In this respect, illness behavior related to a socially unacceptable and nondiscussed disease is clearly different to more acceptable disorders: it is improbable, then, that somaticization is an index of psychological disturbance in the case of sexually transmitted diseases, as it may be in other illness, because of their social unacceptability and consequent lack of secondary gain.

On the other hand, the data in Table 11.2 illustrate that when compared with Illness Behavior Questionnaire norms for a general practice in the same city (Pilowsky and Spence 1983), sexually transmitted disease clinic attenders have in the case of males significantly higher scores on General Hypochondriasis, Affective Inhibition, and Affective Disturbance. Females follow the same trend for General Hypochondriasis, and in comparison on the Whiteley Index of Hypochondriasis with nonpsychiatric patients with malignant disease. They are, however, also lower than the general practice population on Irritability. A general practice population was used for comparison because norms were already available and because a general practice population would provide a comparison with patients with generally mild illness that could be dealt with on an out-patient basis. These data suggest that the sexually transmitted disease clinic population may be closer to a psychiatric population than to a general practice one. Such a suggestion has been made previously by Catalan et al. (1981) who found that 40 percent of the population attending a similar clinic in the United Kingdom scored above the cutoff point on a screening measure for identification of psychiatric cases. Thus while it is apparent that these data may also reflect the fact that the sample has a degree of psychological disturbance, most clearly associated with higher partner numbers (as has been previously demonstrated by Ross 1984), it is probably not advisable to extend these findings to a private practice sexually transmitted disease population who may possibly differ substantially in degree of psychological adjustment.

Nevertheless, it is clear that increasing illness behavior is associated with increasing numbers of sexually transmitted infections and with increasing partner numbers. It is therefore important to recognize that illness behavior in new versus repeating patients is likely to be different, and that clinical response to new patients should include the awareness that their perception of the problem may not be a medical one. At the other end of the spectrum, repeat attenders are most likely to recognize that their behavior is a contributor to their infection and to attribute a much greater degree of meaning (and of illness behavior) to the episode of infection. Counseling repeat attenders about avoidance of risks for infection is thus more likely to be acceptable than counseling of new patients.

DIFFERENCES BETWEEN HOMOSEXUAL AND HETEROSEXUAL MEN

The data in Table 11.4 reveal, interestingly, that there are few differences in illness behavior between homosexual and heterosexual men. Homosexual men are more likely to have higher affective inhibition (which indicates difficulty in expressing personal feelings, especially negative ones, to other people), and a lower Whitely Index of Hypochondriasis. This indicates a lower degree of bodily preoccupation, lower disease phobia and less paranoia toward medical personnel, and less depression.

These data are suggestive of two main differences between homosexual and heterosexual men who attend public STD clinics. First, homosexual men appear to be much more reticent to discuss personal issues with others, including attending medical personnel. From a clinical point of view, this suggests that it may be helpful to encourage such discussion in homosexual men since it is less likely that they will volunteer information on or concerns about personal issues on their own. Given that most homosexuals, because of the degree of stigmatization of their sexuality, are rarely able to discuss personal issues with others (indeed, many may not even acknowledge to others

TABLE 11.4 Differences Between Homosexual and Heterosexual Men in Illness
Behavior

	Heterosexual	Homosexual
General Hypochondriasis	2.8±2.2	3.0±2.3
Disease Conviction	1.9±1.1	1.8±1.3
Psychological vs Somatic Conviction	2.1±0.8	2.2±0.6
Affective Inhibition	2.7±1.2	3.4±1.3+
Affective Disturbance	2.5±1.5	2.9±1.8
Depression	3.1±1.4	2.4±1.4+
Irritability	2.4±1.5	2.1±1.4*
Whiteley Index of Hypochondriasis	4.8±3.3	2.9±2.0*

+p < .075
*p < .05

that they are homosexual) nonjudgmental encouragement may
be appropriate. It is not hard to see why homosexual men
may have more difficulty in discussing interpersonal issues
of concern with others when it is realized that this may
constitute an important defense mechanism to avoid labeling
or stigmatization as homosexual in an antagonistic society.
    Second, the lower level of hypochondriasis in homo-
sexual men (at least, prior to any AIDS cases being notified
in South Australia) confirms the hypothesis that homosexual
men are less preoccupied with health issues and that there
is probably less guilt or venereoneurosis in homosexual
clinic attenders. This finding does suggest that homosexual
men are less concerned at STD infection and probably more
likely to underplay the illness and its impact. There are
probably two reasons for this. First, homosexual men are
usually made much more aware of STD infections through
gay publications and through media reports (particularly
with the advent of AIDS). Second, homosexual men tend to
define themselves in sexual terms (the very name, homosexual, defines them as having sex with persons of the
same gender). Defining oneself in sexual terms makes
STDs much more acceptable as a risk of ones central status, whereas heterosexual men would seldom define themselves as "heterosexual," but rather take their sexual
orientation for granted. To the heterosexual man, therefore, an STD is likely to be of much greater concern and
more unexpected. The unexpected nature of an STD infection will therefore lead to greater concern with one's

state of health than if STD infection is regarded as a probable risk. This would appear to explain the higher level of depression in the heterosexual men. Table 11.5 reports on the correlations between demographic variables and position on the Kinsey Scale. The three significant correlations reveal that homosexual patients are likely to be older than heterosexuals, have higher partner numbers, and to have had more previous STD diagnoses than the heterosexuals. These last two findings are not unexpected, and it is also reasonable to anticipate that homosexual men would be older since heterosexual men tend to marry (and thus usually reduce numbers of sexual partners) by their mid-twenties, thus biasing the sample.

TABLE 11.5 Correlations Between Kinsey Scale Position[a] and Presentation Variables

Variable	Correlation
Age	.30**
Partner Numbers	.22*
Number of Previous STD Diagnoses	.35**

[a]Kinsey Scale is heterosexual = 0 to homosexual = 6
*p < .05
**p < .01

In general, these data do suggest that illness behaviors, at least in the case of sexually transmitted diseases, develop as a function of the number of infections and as the relationship between behavior and infection becomes clear. The meaning of the infection as being an illness is thus probably reinforced by its association with patterns of behavior (such as increased partner numbers) that would not occur with isolated or chance infection. It may therefore be the case that illness behavior in chance as against repeated reinfections with acute conditions, and in socially acceptable versus socially unacceptable illnesses, has different meanings and may serve different psychological functions. However, there is little evidence that illness behavior in homosexual and heterosexual men is markedly different, and it must be concluded that, with the exceptions noted, similar approaches may be used.

12

Psychoimmunology in Homosexual Men

The importance of immune function in both the infection process and the response to infection is sufficiently well established to require little comment. What is less well established is the role that psychological factors play in the competence of the immune system. As far back as 1935, Fleck (1935/1979) commented that belief in the cause of STD infection had moved from the causative organism to emphasis on cofactors and to the concept of carriers and of silent infection. Such cofactors were then, as now, not well understood, but Fleck makes it clear that such cofactors were the only way the variability of susceptibility to and infection with pathogens could be explained given the lack of correspondence between exposure and infection. The recent advent of acquired immune deficiency syndrome (AIDS) has already focused a great deal of attention on variables that affect the body's attack and defense systems, and among the theories put forward to account, to some degree, for the susceptibility of homosexual men to AIDS is that the additional psychological stresses of a homosexual lifestyle and the associated stigma depress immune function. Such a relative immunodepression would thus make the body more susceptible to pathogens and curtail its immediate defense.

In reviewing the literature on the relationship between immune function and psychosocial contributors, Jemmott and Locke (1984) note that there has been for some time clear evidence that recent life stress leads to greater degeneration of overall health: they also note, however, the difficulties surrounding the definition and interpretation of the word "stress" in various studies. While most of the empirical evidence of stress depressing immune function comes from animal studies, there is not as much consistency as might be hoped for in terms of results. Jemmott and Locke report that while most animal studies show that experimental stress has immunosuppressive effects, some have obtained results that suggest that stress may enhance immune function. More specifically, Palmblad (1981), reviewing the temporal sequence of stressor and antigen exposure, has noted that exposure of animals to stress leads to initial depression of investigated immune function, followed by immunostimulation. Looking in detail at the timing, there is increased morbidity or mortality if the microorganism or antigen is administered prior to, or simultaneous with, the exposure to the stressor. On the other hand, an *increased* resistance may be found if the stressor *precedes* the exposure to the antigen. Palmblad suggests that the best interpretation of these data is that stressor exposure may depress host defense as long as it prevails, but thereafter a period of enhanced resistance may follow. Monjan (1981) reports that it is the cellular, rather than the humoral, limb of the immune system that is most affected by states of stress, particularly the heterogeneous groups of cells that comprise the T-cell population.

Psychological factors have also been shown to directly affect immune response. Ader and Cohen (1981), in a series of elegant studies using rats, were able to show consistent immunosuppression as measured by hemagglutinating antibody assays to a conditioned taste stimulus when that taste stimulus had initially been paired with an immunosuppressant agent. They have suggested that the mechanism for this may be adrenocortically mediated, conditioned elevation in steriod levels, but subsequent studies that examined this hypothesis (Ader and Cohen 1981) provided no support for an adrenocortical mediation of conditioned immunosuppression. However, the classical conditioning of immunosuppressive response has been shown to have generalizability across species, across antigens, and across responses, and is independently reproducible. The magnitude of the effect, and the consistency of the response, is compelling evidence for psychological mediation of immune response.

More recently, Blalock (1984) has hypothesized that the immune system may function as part of a reciprocal feedback loop of the nervous system, and that future research may uncover the mechanisms involved. Blalock's suggestion appears to confirm that there are clearly a number of pathways in which psychological and neural events may modify the immune system, and to go further and to suggest that there may also be a reciprocal feedback with the immune system having the ability to influence neural processes. While much of this speculation requires empirical investigation, it is abundantly clear that any specific hypothesis linking psychological variables to immune status has a great deal of suggestive evidence to recommend it.

Several hypotheses may thus be derived for empirical test. First, that immediate stressful conditions (which include stress, anxiety and depression) will lead to decreased mitogenesis and decreased T-cell numbers. Second, that stressful situations in the past (such as parental rearing patterns that homosexual men experienced as children) will also have a similar effect on mitogenesis and T-cell numbers. These two hypotheses by no means cover the major range of operational hypotheses, but are sufficient to demonstrate that psychological variables do have an effect on immune status in homosexual men.

SAMPLE AND METHOD

The sample of South Australian homosexual men was used to test the hypotheses that mood states and parental rearing patterns, as measures of present psychological state and past psychological stresses, will affect mitogenesis and T-cell numbers. Measure of mood state was the Profile of Mood States (POMS) of McNair, Lorr and Droppleman (1971), which measures seven present mood states: anger-hostility, vigor-activity, friendliness, confusion, depression-rejection, tension-anxiety, and fatigue-inertia. Three eight-point semantic differential scales measuring degrees of depression, anxiety, and stress over the past three months were also included. Parental rearing patterns were measured by the EMBU measure (Perris et al. 1980, Ross, Campbell and Clayer 1982, Ross, Clayer and Campbell 1983), and the 14 subscales for maternal and for paternal rearing patterns further factor analyzed (Ross, Campbell and Clayer 1982) to produce three superfactors for each parent: Factor 1 (rejecting and shaming mother or father), Factor 2 (accepting and stimulating mother or father), and Factor 3 (overinvolved and overprotective mother or father). These three superfactors were used as the independent variables rather than the 28 subscales for mother and father together.

Measures of mitogenesis included pokeweed mitogen 1 (a

T-cell dependent B-cell mitogen), concanavalin A 50 (a T- and B-cell mitogen) and phytohemagglutinin 100 (a T-cell mitogen), and measures of T-cell numbers were limited to total T cells, and T-helper, and T-suppressor subsets.

Lymphocyte proliferation

The PBMC were isolated on Ficoll-paque, and cultured at a concentration of $5x10^5$/ml in medium composed of RPMI-1640 supplemented with 10% heat-inactivated fetal bovine serum (CSL Australia), 2 mM glutamine, 100 units/ml penicillin and 100 µg/ml streptomycin. All cultures were set up in microtiter trays, with each well containing 200 µl of the cell suspension and 25 µl of either the mitogen to be tested or culture medium. The cells were incubated at 37°C in a CO_2 incubator. DNA synthesis was measured by adding 25 µl of methyl[^{3}H]-thymidine (Radiochemical Centre, Amersham, England), containing 0.4 µCi, to each well after 68 hours culture. Following a further four-hour incubation, the PBMC were collected onto glass fiber disks using a cell harvester and the disks were then counted in a beta coun- ter. The results are reported as the mean counts per minute of quadruplicate cultures. The stimulation index was calculated as the ratio of the counts per minute in the mitogen stimulated to the unstimulated control cultures.

T-cell numbers were assessed by standard fluorescence assay with monoclonal antibodies OKT-3 (total T-cell num- bers), OKT-4 (T-helpers) and OKT-8 (T-suppressors) and measured by a fluorescence-activated cell sorter.

Data analysis consisted of dividing results on the three mitogens and on the three T-cell categories into quintiles and carrying out one-way analyses of variance on the independent variables across these five groups.

RESULTS AND DISCUSSION

Results are presented in Table 12.1 and Figures 12.1 to 12.4. Looking first at the relationship of parental rearing patterns to mitogenesis, from Figures 12.1–12.3 it can be seen that a consistent pattern emerges. With only two exceptions, the pattern that is exemplified by the mitogen concanavalin A is repeated with the two other mitogens, pokeweed mitogen and phytohemagglutinin. The negative parental rearing patterns give a U-shaped curvilinear relationship with level of mitogenesis, suggesting that those individuals with both the highest *and* the lowest levels of mitogenesis had had very rejecting or very nonrejecting paternal rearing styles. The same pattern, but in this case an *n*-shaped curve, held for the measure of sympathetic and warm paternal parental rearing patterns, again suggesting that the highest *and* lowest mitogenesis was the result of the extremes of parental rearing styles. Maternal curves followed the same pattern as the paternal curves. There appeared to be no consistent relationship between overinvolved parents of either gender and mitogenesis.

TABLE 12.1 Immunological Indices in South Australian Homosexual Men

	Mean	Standard Error
Total T cells (%)	67.1	1.9
Helper T cells (%)	40.1	1.5
Suppressor T cells (%)	15.6	1.4
Con A 50, 72 hours	34,440.4	2,328.0
Pokeweed mitogen, 72 hours	14,108.3	1,293.0
Phytohemagglutinin, 72 hours	38,140.3	2,577.6

These data may offer some important preliminary insights into the nature of distant stressors and their impact on immune competence as measured by mitogenesis. The relative consistency of the pattern across the three mitogens would appear to rule out random effects, as would the relative consistency between maternal and paternal measures. If, as these data show, both very positive and very negative parental rearing patterns predict both high and low levels of mitogenesis, then it could be suggested that each is a stressor. That is, the very positive parental rearing pattern could be seen as producing stress through not sensitizing the individual to stresses that they will have to cope with later in life. Similarly, a very negative parental rearing pattern may have the effect of oversensitizing the individual to environmental stresses.

Thus the apparently "distant" effect of parental rearing patterns may in fact act through its determination of current stress. A second point of major interest is that these data demonstrate that extremes of parental rearing patterns may lead to high or low mitogenesis, without any indication of which leads to which. This does imply that there are at least two distinct groups of individuals who will react either

Figure 12.1   Con A and Parental Rearing Patterns

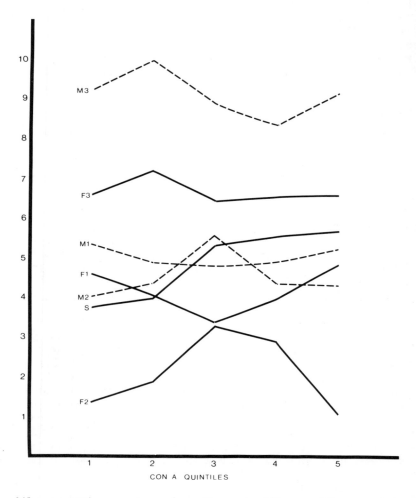

M1, negative maternal patterns; M2, positive maternal patterns; M3, overinvolved maternal patterns; F1, negative paternal patterns; F2, positive paternal patterns; F3, overinvolved paternal patterns; and S, stress.

with increased or decreased mitogenesis to the same stressor. However, the relationship is not a simple one, since for both concanavalin A and pokeweed mitogen stress over the past three months has a linear relationship with mito-

Figure 12.2   Pokeweed Mitogen (PWM) and Parental Rearing Patterns

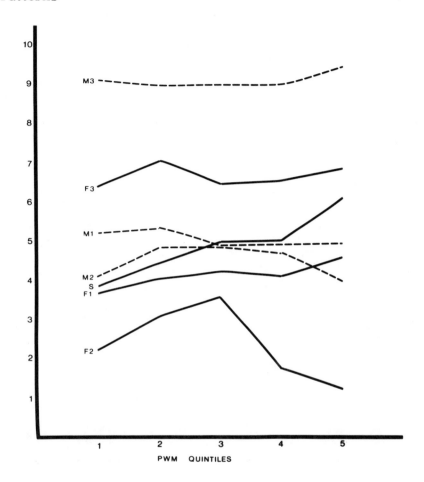

M1, negative maternal patterns; M2, positive maternal patterns; M3, overinvolved maternal patterns; F1, negative paternal patterns; F2, positive paternal patterns; F3, overinvolved paternal patterns; and S, stress.

genesis, with greater stress leading to increased mito-genesis. There was no statistically significant relationship between stress and phytohemagglutinin, so no curve is shown for this.

There are some data that may provide an explanation for these findings. Locke et al. (1979) as reported by

Figure 12.3   Phytohemagglutinin (PHA) and Parental Rearing Patterns

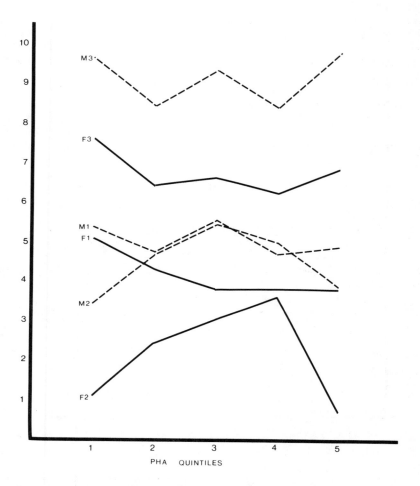

PHA   QUINTILES

M1, negative maternal patterns; M2, positive maternal patterns; M3, overinvolved maternal patterns; F1, negative paternal patterns; F2, positive paternal patterns; F3, overinvolved paternal patterns; and S, stress.

Jemmott and Locke (1984) measured self-reported life-stress changes during intervals of the past year, month, and fortnight in conjunction with swine flu inoculation. They found that only stressful events recorded as having occurred in the past fortnight were related, in a curvilinear fashion, to antibody titer. Antibody response was almost three times greater among those with moderate life stress in this fortnight than among those reporting high or low life-stress change for the same period. These data reported by Locke et al. (1979) provide confirmation that it is the extremes of stress which appear to compromise immune response. At this stage, it would seem a reasonable working hypothesis to suggest that lack of stress may either fail to provide the immunostimulation that may follow stress-related immunosuppression (Palmblad 1981) or be related to the stress at a psychological level being experienced as more acute when it is an unusual event to which the individual has not been sensitized. As an example of this latter point, a moderate stressor may appear major to an individual who has been relatively shielded from stress. On the other hand, a moderate stressor may also appear major to an individual who has suffered previous major stresses and has become sensitized to stress. It must be noted, however, that in the present sample at least, stress over the past three months appears to have a linear relationship with mitogenesis by enhancing it. While discussion of potential mechanisms is beyond the scope of this chapter, we are able to demonstrate a clear and consistent relationship between T-cell mitogenesis and parental rearing patterns. These data do demonstrate that psychological factors distant to measurements of immune function do influence, directly or indirectly, immune function and thus by implication susceptibility to, and response to, infection with pathogens, which may include STDs.

The relationship of immediate mood states to immune functioning provides an opportunity to assess the effect of the immediate psychological environment on cellular immunity. Figure 12.4 illustrates the relationship of the so-called "suppressor" T-cell numbers to mood states as measured on the POMS, self-esteem as measured on the Rosenberg Self-Esteem scale and on the Homosexual Self-Esteem scale (Appendix 3), as well as the 8-point semantic differential scales measuring stress, anxiety, and depression over the past three months.

Initially, total T-cell numbers (the OKT-3 defined subset), helper T cells (the OKT-4 defined subset) and suppressor T cells (the OKT-8 defined subset) were all measured and analyzed by one-way analysis of variance after dividing them into quintiles, with total T-cell numbers and subset numbers as the dependent variable. However, there were no significant associations between helper T-cell numbers and the independent variables, and the patterns of significant differences were almost identical for total T cells

Figure 12.4 T-suppressor Numbers and Mood States

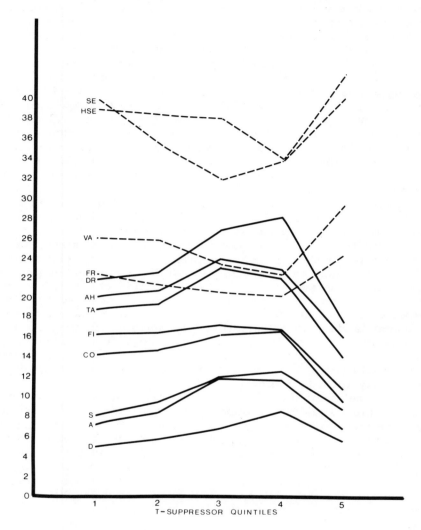

SE, Self-esteem; HSE, Homosexual self-esteem; VA, Vigor-Activity; FR, Friendliness; DR, Depression; AH, Anger-Hostility; TA, Tension-Anxiety; FI, Fatigue; CO, Confusion; S, Stress past 3 months; A, Anxiety past 3 months; and D, Depression past 3 months.

and suppressor T cells, strongly suggesting that it is the suppressor T-cells that account for the differences in total

T-cell numbers. For this reason, suppressor T-cell numbers are presented as the variable best illustrating the relationship between mood state and other psychological states and immune function. Reference to Figure 12.4 shows as in Figures 12.1–12.3, a remarkably consistent and curvilinear relationship between suppressor T-cell numbers and the seven mood states measured by the POMS. Of particular interest is the fact that the positive mood states (vigor-activity, friendliness) and the two measures of self-esteem, both general and homosexual self-esteem, all show a similar U-shaped curvilinear curve, which suggests that both low and high suppressor T-cell numbers are associated with increased positive mood states and self-esteem. The converse curvilinear relationship, an n-shaped curve, occurs not only in the negative mood states (depression, anger-hostility, tension-anxiety, fatigue-inertia, confusion) but also with the three semantic differential measures of stress, anxiety, and depression over the past 12 months. These reversed curves also imply that it is the lower levels of negative mood states that are associated with both high and low suppressor T-cell numbers, and as with the mitogenic response study previously described, this would also imply that stress itself is not directly related to these affects, but that perhaps two or more processes are operating. These processes may relate to the hypothesis that the particularly low levels of negative mood states may be caused by overcompensation and thus also be stress related: however, this seems an unlikely explanation.

Greene et al. (1978) also used the POMS to study the relationship between self-reported life stress and immune functioning in young people inoculated with the Victoria flu virus. They found that subjects who were higher in life-change stress and who also had a higher POMS vigor score had lower lymphoctye cytotoxicity and hemagglutination-inhibition antibody titers. These results, at least with regard to the vigor score, are consistent with the present findings. A second study that used the POMS, that of Locke and Heisel (1977), found no relationship between mood state and antibody response during immunization.

These data nevertheless demonstrate that immediate mood states and self-esteem, as well as stress, anxiety, and depression over the past three months, are associated with suppressor T-cell numbers; however, the association is clearly not a simple one given the nonlinear association between the dependent and independent variables. It is possible that other factors may be intervening to produce the relationships demonstrated, and that the association between mood states and suppressor T-cell numbers is not direct. Nevertheless, it is important to note that Rose (1980) has reported that cortisol and catecholamine secretion rates may increase in intensely pleasurable situations as well as stressful ones. It is quite likely that our mood state findings are related to this rather than to stress as the mediating variable in both T-cell mitogenesis and T-cell numbers. It is also interesting to speculate that some of these variations of immune function in active homosexual men may be due not to lifestyle-related stresses but to the hedonistically related cortisol or catecholamine excretion of a "fast-lane" lifestyle.

On the other hand, chronic physical stress has been associated with enhanced immunocompetence (Monjan 1981) whereas acute physical stress is associated with diminished immune function. Clearly, in this chapter we are not in a position to discuss the mediation pathways associated with the present data. Given the consistent and significant associations between both distant psychological events (parental rearing patterns experienced) and lymphocyte proliferation and mood state and T-cell numbers, however, we can clearly conclude that there is a consistent and demonstrable relationship between psychological factors and immune functioning in homosexual men.

CONCLUSIONS

In conclusion, we can confirm that psychological variables have an influence on immune function in homosexual men. From the literature and the present data, it is reasonable to assume that psychological status will affect STD infection through modification of the susceptibility of the individual to infection after inoculation by various pathogens.

It is not, however, possible to go beyond this knowledge at this point in time. In his foreword to Ader (1981), Good writes that while he knows, as an immunologist, that attitudes, states of mind, grief, depression or anxiety may influence the body's defenses, he is left with a feeling of inadequacy because he is unable to tell how they work. In this chapter, a similar conclusion must be reached. Nevertheless, in considering the influence of psychosocial factors on STD infection, we must also consider that these influences occur not only at the level of determining behavior, but also at the level of potential determination of disease outcome, or indeed whether infection establishes itself at all. Thus at an organic, as well as a behavioral level, psychosocial variables play a central part in influencing contraction of, and course of, STD infections.

13

Conclusions and Models for Future Research

In the research reported in this book, we commenced with a number of assumptions that there was nothing intrinsically abnormal about a homosexual orientation, and that a large proportion of the variance of STD infections would be accountable for by social and psychological variables. Both of these assumptions have been demonstrated. First, it is apparent that while some subsets of a homosexual lifestyle may have negative connotations, others may have positive ones in the same way as a heterosexual orientation has both positive and negative connotations. These connotations, it is also clear, will depend to a large degree on the individual and his interpretation of and adjustment to his social and interpersonal milieu.

Second, it has been possible to demonstrate that both social and psychological variables are consistently implicated in the three aspects of sexual behavior that we have selected as determining levels of STD infection: partner numbers, particular sexual practices, and places of partner contact. While there are clearly interactions between these three aspects, in each we find that social variables such as culture, degree of socialization into the homosexual subculture, societal reaction to homosexuality, age of homosexual identification and activity, education, religious belief, and beliefs about social sex roles in the individual, are implicated. Other variables that refer to psychological state, such as parental rearing patterns experienced, mood states, levels of stress, anxiety and depression, self-esteem, sex-role conservatism, and self-rating on a number of dimensions as well as social sex role behavior, are also implicated. The patterns that emerge are consistent across cultures and in replicates taken some time apart, and we are thus able to be certain to a greater degree that what has been demonstrated is not statistical artifact. Particular patterns, of course, are referred to in the chapters that specifically deal with various aspects of sexual behaviors that may determine STD infection.

Partner preferences have also emerged as a potentially important variable in determining the risk of STD infection, and clearly a greater level of research into this area is warranted. However, it is also apparent that there is a significant degree of chance in STD infection, and that we will never be able to satisfactorily explain all the variance attributable to STD infection.

Implicit in what has been described above is a model of behavioral influences on STD infection, and this model is illustrated in Table 13.1. We assume that temporally, an individual first attends a locale where potential sexual partners may congregate; partner(s) are then approached, and particular sexual practices will then occur. However, good cases could be made for other temporal arrangements, and the diagram in Table 13.1 is oversimplified to provide single paths only from one variable and one temporal level to another. Unstandardized regression weights have been used because the intention is to show only the relative weightings of *linear* interactions in this model. It will also be clear from the body of this book that a great many of the relationships between the variables we have investigated are *curvilinear* and thus would produce correlations approximating zero: for this reason also, the model is illustrative only of some implicit assumptions and not of its success in predicting outcome assuming linear relationships between variables. However, if we are to fully understand the relationships between sexual behavior and STD infections, we must commence from the point of basic models and modify or replace them.

Much of the present work, however, has concentrated not on the antecedents of STD infection but the psychological sequelae. Such sequelae will depend to a great extent on the meaning of sexuality, homosexuality, and STD infection to the individual, and we will have little success in treating individuals or helping them to reduce risks unless we understand that there will be a range of reactions to STD infection and that our behavior as clinicians will need to be based on our perception of the meaning of his sexuality and his infection to the patient. For this

TABLE 13.1 Unstandardized Regression Weights between Variables in STD Infection Model for South Australian Homosexual Men

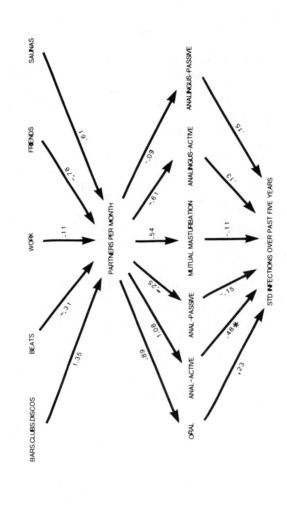

* p < .05

reason, an appreciation of the multiple meanings of sexually related diseases and the multiple meanings of sexuality and homosexuality to the patient is critical, as is an understanding of illness behavior as it applies to STD infection.

In clinician-patient interactions, one of the most downplayed aspects is of course the clinician, and unless we realize that the outcome of the treatment will depend as much on us as on the patient, we are doomed to continue painful and ineffective consultations. The range of attitudes to sexuality, homosexuality, and STD infections outlined will also occur in physicians and nursing staff, and to the extent that they explicitly or implicitly intrude, will defeat the goal of effective and empathic treatment. These attitudes will include political and social beliefs as well as reactions to particular behaviors or individuals. Nor are researchers exempt, as I have hopefully managed to convey the message that even research formulations will contain implicit assumptions about the nature of homosexuality and STDs. We will all continue to make implicit assumptions, but it is preferable that we recognize and state these to enable proper assessment of our work.

Finally, we cannot afford to ignore the fact that psychological variables will determine not only sexual behaviors but also affect somatic functioning through the immune system. While the mechanisms that underlie these effects are not clearly understood, a potentially critical aspect of venereology is to develop an appreciation of the factors that determine whether an infection becomes established or is controlled by the body's defense mechanisms. We all recognize that there is a large gap in our understanding of why one inoculation with a potential pathogen does not equal one infection, and some of the evidence presented here may help to explain some of the factors involved in psychoimmunological terms.

It will also be obvious that psychovenereology is still in its infancy, and that a great deal of further research is both necessary and possible. If I were to highlight areas of particular importance, they would be psychoimmunology and the nature, dimensionality, and etiology of sexual attitudes. Clearly, it is necessary to move one step behind sexual behaviors to the attitudes that underlie them, and the occurrence of two or three attitudes consistently with sexual practices, partner numbers, and the frequenting of particular locales for sexual partners, suggests some common underlying dimensions. Further research would be valuable in this area. Nor must we ignore the interactions that will occur between attitudes and behaviors, despite the complexity of some of the statistical models involved.

The bottom line of the success of this book, however, will be its applied usefulness to clinicians as they attempt to understand and effectively treat homosexual men with STD infections. Given the major risks involved in STD infections with the appearance of AIDS, modification of high-risk activities to lower risk levels is important, and if this can be done with an understanding of the dynamics involved in drives toward particular sexual behaviors, then it will have a greater chance of success, and less of an aura of enforced change. No modification of health risks can succeed unless the individual at risk has insight into the determinants of risk-related behaviors, and has an integral involvement in an attempt to reduce those risks: if this work helps provide such insight, it will hopefully be justified in terms of individual development as well as of risk reduction. Ultimately, however, we can agree with Hart's comment of over a decade ago that STDs are a behavioral problem that require focus on the individual and his social environment, and attempt to move beyond this to an understanding of the forces involved.

Appendixes

1

The Four-Country Questionnaire

UNIVERSITY OF MELBOURNE
Department of Psychology

UNIVERSITY OF STOCKHOLM
Psychological Laboratories

RESEARCH SURVEY OF SOCIAL FACTORS AND THE MALE HOMOSEXUAL

    This questionnaire is part of a cross-cultural piece of research which
is designed to examine the social and cultural factors which affect
homosexuals in different societies which have different legal and social
attitudes toward homosexuality. It consists of a series of questions and
of psychometric scales, particularly designed so that they can be compared
statistically across societies. Some of these scales will have special
instructions, which you should read carefully before commencing to score
them. In general, because this is a relatively long questionnaire, we
suggest that the best idea is to put the first response that comes into
your head, and not to think a long time about items: not only has it been
found that the first response is the most accurate, but if you think too
much about some of the items, you may decide that it is impossible to
answer them accurately. If this happens, go back and put your first,
general response to the question as it applies to you. Almost all the
questions require only that you mark a scale or a box with √ or X, or
circle a letter (see examples below). The questionnaire is anonymous. You
will find with it a stamped addressed envelope: please post the
questionnaire when completed, if possible within a week or two of receiving
it.

Here are examples of the 3 ways to mark the scales:

    - Mark the space at the right of the appropriate response e.g., X
    - Circle the appropriate letter. (If absolutely uncertain, circle ?).
      Y = yes, N = no, A = agree, D = disagree (as it applies to you), e.g.
      A D, or Y ? N
    - On the scales, there is a word at each end of the scale and the
      subject at the left of the same line which you must rate. If you
      felt, in the following example, that your cat was very happy, you
      would put √ close to the Happy end of the scale. In some cases, you

are also asked to rate yourself on the same scale: If you felt that you were somewhat sad, you would put X at the appropriate point. e.g.,

Cat   Happy   Sad

/ √ /   /   /   / X /

Any other responses are explained as they occur in the questionnaire. Your cooperation is strongly appreciated.

Age _____ City of residence _____ Education (years) ____
Occupation _____ Religion: Practising ___, Normal ___, None ___
                       (If practising, specify which) _____
Social level of Parents:
Class 1 ("upper")   ___
Class 2 ("middle")   ___
Class 3 ("working") ___
Would you describe yourself as:

Exclusively   Predominantly   More Homosexual   Equally Homosexual
Homosexual ___   Homosexual ___   than Heterosexual ___ and Heterosexual ___
      More Heterosexual   Predominantly   Exclusively
      than Homosexual ___   Heterosexual ___   Heterosexual ___

How long since you became actively homosexual? ___ (years)
How long before that did you realise that you were homosexual? ___ (years)
Have you ever been married to a woman? Y N Have you been engaged? Y N
If Y to above, are you: Still married ___ Separated, Divorced, Widowed ___
At what age did you marry? ___ Did (or does) your wife know of your
homosexuality? Y ? N

How do you think the following people would react (or have reacted) to your homosexuality? If they know and have reacted, put X on the scale at the appropriate point. Otherwise, put √ for the way you think they would react.

	Accept				Reject		Accept				Reject
Mother	/	/	/	/	/	Father	/	/	/	/	/	
Brother	/	/	/	/	/	Sister	/	/	/	/	/	
Aunts	/	/	/	/	/	Uncles	/	/	/	/	/	
Best heterosexual friend (same sex)	/	/	/	/	/	Best heterosexual friend (opp. sex)	/	/	/	/	/	
Teachers	/	/	/	/	/	Ministers of religion	/	/	/	/	/	
Grandparents	/	/	/	/	/	Work Associates	/	/	/	/	/	
Other people at work	/	/	/	/	/	Your boss	/	/	/	/	/	
Neighbours	/	/	/	/	/	Heterosexuals in general	/	/	/	/	/	
Customers or clients	/	/	/	/	/	Friends of parents	/	/	/	/	/	
Most other heterosexual friends (same sex)	/	/	/	/	/	Most other heterosexual friends (opp. sex)	/	/	/	/	/	

From how many heterosexuals do you try to conceal your homosexuality?
(Circle the appropriate response). All   Most   Some   Few   None

Would there be problems at work if people found out? Yes   Some   Few   None
Has (or would) being labelled Homosexual bother you? Yes   No

Do you think people are likely to break off a social relationship with
someone they think is homosexual? All   Most   Half   Some   None

Do you think people are likely to make life difficult for someone they
think is homosexual? All   Most   Half   Some   None

	Accept				Reject
How do you think most people feel about homosexuals?	/	/	/	/	/

For the following questions, please circle A (agree) or D (disagree).

Homosexuality could best be described as an illness.	A	?	D
Homosexuals and heterosexuals are basically different in more ways than sexual preference.	A	?	D
There is nothing immoral about being a homosexual.	A	?	D
What consenting adults do in private is nobody's business, as long as they don't hurt other people.	A	?	D
It would not bother me if I had children who were homosexual.	A	?	D
A person is born homosexual or heterosexual.	A	?	D
There's nothing one can do to make oneself more or less homosexual.	A	?	D
I have a number of good qualities.	A	?	D
I am inclined to feel that I'm a failure.	A	?	D
I have harder time than other people in gaining friends.	A	?	D
I often feel downcast and dejected.	A	?	D
I feel that I have a lot to be proud of.	A	?	D

How much do you think homosexuality violates the following?

	A Lot			Not at All	
Conventional Morality	/	/	/	/	/
Religious (Christian) Morality	/	/	/	/	/
Conformity in General	/	/	/	/	/

Up to adolescence, how well did you get on personally with each parent?

	Well			Not Well	
Mother	/	/	/	/	/
Father	/	/	/	/	/

How much influence did each of the following sources have on your behavior?

	Strong			Weak	
Father	/	/	/	/	/
Mother	/	/	/	/	/
Male friends of your own age	/	/	/	/	/

Female friends your own age   / / / / /
Teachers or school   / / / / /
_____ Other sources (specify)   / / / / /

How old were you when you realised that some people think that
homosexuality was wrong, deviant or different? ___

What did you see as being the main difference between men and women at that
time? (Specify) _____

Below are a series of scales. To the left appear a number of individuals or
statements. Rate each on the four scales as it appears to you with an X.

When you first became active   Happy   / / / / / Sad
homosexually, did you think of   Active   / / / / / Passive
yourself as: Strong   / / / / / Weak
   Masculine   / / / / / Feminine

How do you think of yourself now: Strong   / / / / / Weak
   Passive   / / / / / Active
   Happy   / / / / / Sad
   Masculine   / / / / / Feminine

Ideally, you would like to be: Passive   / / / / / Active
   Sad   / / / / / Happy
   Feminine   / / / / / Masculine
   Weak   / / / / / Strong

How do you think of homosexual men: Masculine   / / / / / Feminine
   Weak   / / / / / Strong
   Active   / / / / / Passive
   Happy   / / / / / Sad
   Passive   / / / / / Active

How do you think of heterosexual   Feminine   / / / / / Masculine
women: Strong   / / / / / Weak
   Happy   / / / / / Sad
   Passive   / / / / / Active

In completely homosexual company,   Passive   / / / / / Active
how do you think of yourself: Weak   / / / / / Strong
   Sad   / / / / / Happy
   Feminine   / / / / / Masculine

How do you think of your mother: Weak   / / / / / Strong
   Masculine   / / / / / Feminine
   Happy   / / / / / Sad
   Passive   / / / / / Active

How do you think of your father: Active   / / / / / Passive
   Happy   / / / / / Sad
   Masculine   / / / / / Feminine
   Weak   / / / / / Strong

Below are a series of statements. Indicate by placing an X on the scale the extent to which you agree or disagree with it.

	Agree	Disagree
It is natural for male homosexuals to be more feminine than male heterosexuals.	/ / / / /	
Male homosexuals often act as if they are more feminine than male heterosexuals.	/ / / / /	
Because they prefer men, male homosexuals must like women to some extent.	/ / / / /	
Being homosexual means that one is a third sex, in between males and females.	/ / / / /	
Most people think that male homosexuals are feminine to some extent.	/ / / / /	
Because individuals may think male homosexuals are more feminine than heterosexual males, the homosexual ones tend to act that way.	/ / / / /	
If a man wants to have sex with another man, then he must identify himself to some extent, however small, as a female.	/ / / / /	
Most people only see sexual relationships as being valid between a man and a woman.	/ / / / /	
Most homosexuals tend to imitate the heterosexual world and its values too much.	/ / / / /	
No matter how hard it tries, the homosexual world is going to have to accept and use the values of the heterosexual world.	/ / / / /	

	Frequently	Rarely	1-2 times	No
Have you ever cross-dressed a) As a child	—	—	—	—
b) Since adolescence	—	—	—	—

	Clear	Unclear
With your parents, were the roles of man and woman:	/ / / / /	

	Anti-homosexual	Pro-homosexual
To what extent do you think people in your country are anti-homosexual, compared with other places?	/ / / / /	
	/ / / / /	

From what you've heard or learned about homosexuality,
do you think that boys who do any of the following
are likely to become homosexual? Circle the response
you think is most appropriate.

Played with dolls.	Y	?	N
Played with trucks and blocks.	Y	?	N
Took part in sports.	Y	?	N
Avoided sports.	Y	?	N
Played mostly with boys.	Y	?	N
Played mostly with girls.	Y	?	N
Tended to be a "loner".	Y	?	N

If (or when) you were publicly exposed as homosexual to your family,
friends and the community, how much of the following would (or did) you
feel? Put X if you think you would feel this way, √ if when this happened
you actually felt this.

	A Lot				Not Much

Fear about losing friends. / / / / /

Embarrassment or shame about people seeing
you as a homosexual. / / / / /

Guilt or anxiety about how people would think
of you morally. / / / / /

Worry about how it might affect you getting
on in life. / / / / /

It would make you feel small and lower your
prestige. / / / / /

You would feel that society was punishing you
for being homosexual. / / / / /

Where do you mix most with other homosexual people? Put 1 for the most
important, 2 for the next important, and so on, through the list.

                    Bars and Clubs..........
                    Private gatherings......
                    Beats or conveniences......
                    Gay activist meetings.......
                    Work........
                    Other (specify)...... ...

At present, what proportion of your leisure
time is spent in involvement with the homosexual
subculture (excluding time with people you
live with)?

None / / / / / All

In the year when you first became homosexually   <u>None</u>   <u>All</u>
active, what proportion?   /   /   /   /   /

Do you have a general stereotype of the sort of person you do (or would)
get on best with in a homosexual affair? (i.e., what is your "ideal man"?)
On the following scales, rate where you think <u>you</u> fall with an X, where
your <u>ideal partner</u> would fall with a √ . If the attribute is unimportant,
put the √ in the box at the end.

Emotional	/ / / / / Not Emot.	Tall	/ / / / /	Short
Unconventional	/ / / / / Convent.	Thin	/ / / / /	Fat
Sexy	/ / / / / Not sexy	Hairy	/ / / / /	Smooth
Active	/ / / / / Passive	Clean-shaven	/ / / / /	Facial hair
Introverted	/ / / / / Extroverted	Long hair	/ / / / /	Short hair
Intelligent	/ / / / / Not Intell.	Large penis	/ / / / /	Small penis
Socially involved	/ / / / / Not Involv.	Well-dressed	/ / / / /	Casual
Masculine	/ / / / / Feminine	Rugged	/ / / / /	Delicate
Warm	/ / / / / Cold	Similar Interests	/ / / / /	Dissimilar

When you are having sexual relations with another man, do you prefer:
  (Mark one) Fellatio (insertor)   __   (Mark one) Anal sex (insertor   __
               Fellatio (insertee   __   Anal sex (insertee)   __
               " " " (doesn't   __   " " " (doesn't
               matter which, or both) __   matter which, or both) __

                                           Mutual masturbation   __
                                           Full body contact   __
                                         Anything else (specify)
                                         ....

Have you ever had a homosexual relationship which lasted
for over two years?   Y   N
Have you ever had a heterosexual relationship which lasted
over two years?   Y   N
Are you present in a homosexual relationship that has
lasted over two years?   Y   N
If Y to the first or third questions, please answer the
following: (up to *)
    In your present (or your most successful) relationship, did
    You both work on the basis of roles of any kind? Y   N
  Were these: Sexual only   Y   N   Dominant-submissive   Y   N
               Male-Female   Y   N   Only with domestic tasks Y   N

If these roles exist, do they remain rigid or often change? Rigid   Change
Is your relationship monogamous?   Y   N
*Do you believe that homosexual relationships should occur:
                 Between two people   Y   ?   N

Between more than two, it doesn't matter   Y   ?   N
Homosexual relationships are not natural   Y   ?   N
Homosexual need not form relationships   Y   ?   N

Have you ever had a veneral disease? Please indicate 1) Type, and 2) number of times.

Gonorrhea   Y   N ......   Syphilis   Y   N ......
Other (specify) ....

The last time, did you go to a VD clinic or your general practitioner first?

Clinic __   GP __

Did you admit that the source of infection was homosexual?   Y   N

Have you had any negative experience in a clinic? Y   N   If Y, What .....
....

Did you go to any particular clinic? Y   N   If Y, Why? ....

For each time you got VD: Did you know which individual you got it from (i.e., you didn't have to guess) 1) Y N 2) Y N 3) Y N 4) Y N 5) Y N

Did you know the name, address or any other details so the person could be contacted if necessary? 1) Y N 2) Y N 3) Y N 4) Y N 5) Y N

Taking a typical figure over the last year, how many different partners per month, on average would you have had? ....

Where do you usually meet sexual partners?
(Mark one) Beats __   Bars/Clubs __
Work __   Friends __

To what extent do you think the laws in your country support equality for women, compared with other places? Support /   /   /   / Don't support

To what extent do you think in general believe that women should have equal rights, compared with other places?
Should have /   /   /   / Should't have

Have you ever seen a Psychiatrist: Regarding your homosexuality   Y   N
For any other reason   Y   N

If there is any comment you would care to make or any question you may wish to elaborate on, please do so in the space at the end. When you have finished, place the completed questionnaire in the envelope provided, and mail it as soon as is practical. Thank you for your cooperation in this

research. There are two further rapid scales to be completed which are
attached. You need not do them at the same time if you don't want to, but
please complete them before you post the questionnaire back. No stamp is
required on the envelope.

- - - ° ° ° - - -

The South Australian Questionnaire

I. GENERAL

   1. Date of birth ....

   2. Place of birth ....

   3. Details of visits outside Australia (country, dates to and from):

      ....

      ....

   4. Details of visits to other States (in past 5 years) (city, dates to and from):

      ....

      ....

   5. Education - Primary only .... 1-3 years secondary ....

               Over 3 years secondary .... Tertiary ....

II. SEXUAL

1. Sexual activity	Past year	Past 5 years
(a) exclusively heterosexual	....	....
(b) predominantly heterosexual with some homosexual activity	....	....
(c) bisexual	....	....
(d) predominantly homosexual with some heterosexual activity	....	....
(e) exclusively homosexual	....	....

2. Sexual partners

   (a) abstinent (none) ....

   (b) monogamous (only one) ....

   (c) under 50 per year ....

   (d) 50-100 per year ....

   (e) over 100 per year ....

3. At present, what proportion of your leisure time is spent in involvement with the homosexual subculture (excluding time with people you live with)? Place an X at the appropriate point on the scale:

```
     None     25%      50%      75%      All
      L_____I_____I_____I_____J
```

4. How many different sexual partners, on average per month, would you have had over the last year? ....

5. When you have had sexual relations with another man in the past year, do you have (place an X at any appropriate point on the scales: you may mark as you like):

   (a) Oral sex (partner puts his penis in your mouth, or you put your penis in your partner's mouth)

```
     Never    25%      50%      75%     Always
      L_____I_____I_____I_____J
```

   (b) Anal intercourse (active) (you put your penis in your partner's anus)

```
     Never    25%      50%      75%     Always
      L_____I_____I_____I_____J
```

   (c) Anal intercourse (passive) (your partner puts his penis in your anus)

```
     Never    25%      50%      75%     Always
      L_____I_____I_____I_____J
```

(d) Mutual masturbation

```
Never     25%      50%      75%      Always
  L_____|_____|_____|_____J
```

(e) Oral-Anal sex ("rimming") (active - you put your tongue in your partner's anus)

```
Never     25%      50%      75%      Always
  L_____|_____|_____|_____J
```

(f) Oral-Anal sex (passive - your partner puts his tongue in your anus)

```
Never     25%      50%      75%      Always
  L_____|_____|_____|_____J
```

(g) Anything else (please specify) ....

```
Never     25%      50%      75%      Always
  L_____|_____|_____|_____J
```

6. For how many years have you been homosexually active? ....

7. Where do you usually meet sexual partners? Mark 1 the most important, 2 the next most important, and so on. If you never go to to a place, leave the box opposite it blank.

Bars/Clubs/Discos   _____

Beats   _____

Work   _____

Friends   _____

Sauna   _____

III. DRUG USE	Past year	Past 5 years
Cigarettes (give average per day)	....	....
Alcohol (average days per week	....	....
(average drinks per day)	....	....
Marijuana (average episodes per year)	....	....

	Past year	Past 5 years
Heroin or morphine (average episodes per year)	....	....
Amyl Nitrite ("poppers") (average episodes per year)	....	....
Other (specify)		

IV. BLOOD PRODUCTS

	Past year	Past 5 years
Given blood (average times per year)	....	....
Received blood (total episodes)	....	....
Tattooed (yes/no)	....	....
Hepatitis B vaccine (yes/no)	....	....
Other (specify)		

V. CURRENT SYMPTOMS

	Yes	No
Skin abnormalities	....	....
Shortness of breath	....	....
Cough for more than a week	....	....
Fever for more than a week	....	....
Night sweats	....	....
Diarrhoea for more than a week	....	....
Unintentional weight loss of greater than 10 pounds	....	....
Increased fatigue requiring 1-2 hours more sleep each night	....	....
Diminished sexual drive or urge (loss of libido)	....	....
Difficult or painful swallowing	....	....
Nausea or vomiting	....	....

	Yes	No
Easy bruising or unusual bleeding	....	....

Other (specify) ....

VI. PAST MEDICAL HISTORY

1. Have you been hospitalised or had an operation in past 5 years?

   Date   Details

   ....

   ....

   ....

2. Have you had a serious medical illness in past 5 years?

   Date   Details

   ....

   ....

   ....

3. Have you ever taken any medication on a regular basis for more than one month?

   Details

   ....

   ....

   ....

4. Are you currently taking any medication?

   Details

   ....

5. What specific illnesses have you had in the last twelve months?

   Details

   ....

   ....

   ....

6. Past infections (number of times)

	Past year	Past 5 years
Gonorrhoes - penile	....	....
throat	....	....
anus	....	....
Syphilis	....	....
Hepatitis	....	....
Herpes simplex - lips	....	....
penis	....	....
anus	....	....
Herpes zoster (shingles) or chickenpox	....	....
Warts - penis	....	....
anus	....	....
Non-specific urethritis	....	....
Glandular fever	....	....
Diarrhoea requiring medical attention	....	....

7. Have you ever had a cancer of any kind?

   Details

   ....

8. Have you ever had x-ray or radiation treatment for any condition?

   Details

   ....

9. When did you last have a chest x-ray?

   Date

   ....

VII. STRESS

1. How much stress have you been under in the last couple of months?
   Place an X at the appropriate point on the scale:

   None   A Lot
   L_____|_____|_____|_____J

2. How anxious have you been in the last couple of months? Place an X
   at the appropriate point on the scale:

   Not at all   Always
   anxious   anxious
        L_____|_____|_____J

3. How depressed have you felt in the last couple of months? Place an
   X at the appropriate point on the scale:

   Never   Always
   depressed   depressed
        L_____|_____|_____J

3

The Homosexual
Self-Esteem Scale

1. Homosexuals are usually superior in many ways to nonhomosexuals.
2. Homosexuality may best be described as an illness.
3. I do not care who knows about my homosexuality.
4. I wish I were not homosexual.
5. I would not want to give up my homosexuality even if I could.
6. Homosexuals and heterosexuals are basically different in more ways than simple sexual preference.
7. It would not bother me if I had children who were homosexual.
8. There is nothing immoral about being homosexual.
9. There's nothing one can do to make oneself more or less homosexual.
10. Homosexuality tends to have a negative effect on society at large.
11. Homosexuality may best be described as a mental illness.

4

The Homosexual
Sexual Attitudes Inventory

This questionnaire is anonymous, to encourage truthful answers.

Read each statement carefully, then underline or circle the "yes" (Y) or "no" (N) answer, depending on your views. If you cannot decide, circle the "?" reply. Please answer EVERY question. There are no right or wrong answers. Don't think too long over each question; try to give an immediate answer which represents your FEELING on each issue. Some questions are similar to others; there are good reasons for getting at the same attitude in slightly different ways.

1. Sex without love ('impersonal sex') is highly unsatisfactory.   Y   ?   N
2. Conditions have to be just right to get me excited sexually.   Y   ?   N
3. All in all I am satisfied with my sex life.   Y   ?   N
4. Sometimes it has been a problem to control my sex feelings.   Y   ?   N
5. If I love a person I could do anything with them.   Y   ?   N
6. I get pleasant feeling from touching my sexual parts.   Y   ?   N
7. I have been deprived sexually.   Y   ?   N
8. Sex contacts have never been a problem to me.   Y   ?   N
9. It is disturbing to see necking in public.   Y   ?   N
10. Sexual feelings are sometimes unpleasant to me.   Y   ?   N
11. Something is lacking in my sex life.   Y   ?   N
12. My sex behaviour has never caused me any trouble.   Y   ?   N
13. My love life has been disappointing.   Y   ?   N
14. I have felt guilty about sex experiences.   Y   ?   N
15. At times I have been afraid of myself for what I might do sexually.   Y   ?   N
16. I have strong sex feelings but when I get a chance I can't seem to express myself.   Y   ?   N
17. It doesn't take much to get me excited sexually.   Y   ?   N
18. My parents' influence has inhibited me sexually.   Y   ?   N
19. Thoughts about sex disturb me more than they should.   Y   ?   N
20. There are some things I wouldn't want to do with anyone.   Y   ?   N
21. I get excited sexually very easily.   Y   ?   N
22. The thought of a sex orgy is disgusting to me.   Y   ?   N

23.	I find the thought of a coloured sex partner particularly exciting.	Y	?	N
24.	I like to look at sexy pictures.	Y	?	N
25.	My conscience bothers me too much.	Y	?	N
26.	Sometimes sexual feelings overpower me.	Y	?	N
27.	I feel nervous with the opposite sex.	Y	?	N
28.	Sex thoughts drive me almost crazy.	Y	?	N
29.	When I get excited I can think of nothing else but satisfaction.	Y	?	N
30.	I feel at ease with people of the opposite sex.	Y	?	N
31.	I don't like to be kissed.	Y	?	N
32.	It is hard to talk with people of the opposite sex.	Y	?	N
33.	I enjoy petting.	Y	?	N
34.	I worry a lot about sex.	Y	?	N
35.	Seeing a person nude doesn't interest me.	Y	?	N
36.	Sometimes thinking about sex makes me very nervous.	Y	?	N
37.	Perverted thoughts have sometimes bothered me.	Y	?	N
38.	I am embarrassed to talk about sex.	Y	?	N
39.	Sex jokes disgust me.	Y	?	N
40.	I believe in taking my pleasures where I find them.	Y	?	N
41.	Young people should be allowed out at night without being too closely checked.	Y	?	N
42.	I have sometimes felt like humiliating my sex partner.	Y	?	N
43.	I have been involved with more than one sex affair at the same time.	Y	?	N
44.	I have sometimes felt hostile to my sex partner.	Y	?	N
45.	I like to look at pictures of nudes.	Y	?	N
46.	If I had the chance to see people making love, without being seen, I would take it.	Y	?	N
47.	Pornographic writings should be freely allowed to be published.	Y	?	N
48.	Prostitution should be legally permitted.	Y	?	N
49.	There are too many immoral plays on T.V.	Y	?	N
50.	I had some bad sex experiences when I was young.	Y	?	N
51.	There should be no censorship, on sexual grounds, of plays and films.	Y	?	N
52.	Sex is far and away my greatest pleasure.	Y	?	N
53.	Sexual permissiveness threatens to undermine the entire foundation of civilised society.	Y	?	N
54.	Absolute faithfulness to one partner throughout life is nearly as silly as celibacy.	Y	?	N
55.	I would enjoy watching my usual partner having intercourse with someone else.	Y	?	N
56.	Sex play among young children is quite harmless.	Y	?	N
57.	I would prefer to have a new sex partner every night.	Y	?	N
58.	I prefer partners who are several years older than myself.	Y	?	N

59.	My sexual fantasies often involve flogging.	Y	?	N
60.	I make lots of vocal noises during intercourse.	Y	?	N
61.	There are some things I do to please my sex partner.	Y	?	N
62.	I don't always know for sure when I have had an orgasm.	Y	?	N
63.	To me few things are more important than sex.	Y	?	N
64.	My sex partner satisfies all my physical needs completely.	Y	?	N
65.	Sex is not all that important to me.	Y	?	N
66.	Most men are sex-mad.	Y	?	N
67.	Being good in bed is terribly important to my partner.	Y	?	N
68.	I find it easy to tell my sex partner what I like, or don't like about his love-making.	Y	?	N
69.	I would like my sex partner to be more expert and experienced.	Y	?	N
70.	I sometimes feel like scratching and biting my partner during intercourse.	Y	?	N
71.	I feel sexually less competent than my friends.	Y	?	N
72.	Group sex appeals to me.	Y	?	N
73.	The thought of an illicit relationship excites me.	Y	?	N
74.	I usually feel aggressive with my sexual partner.	Y	?	N
75.	I am afraid of sexual relationships.	Y	?	N
76.	I can't stand people touching me.	Y	?	N
77.	Physical sex is the most important part of marriage.	Y	?	N
78.	Physical attraction is extremely important to me.	Y	?	N
79.	In a sexual union, tenderness is the most important quality.	Y	?	N
80.	Male genitals are aesthetically unpleasing.	Y	?	N
81.	I object to four-letter swear words being used in mixed company.	Y	?	N
82.	I cannot discuss sexual matters with my habitual sex partner.	Y	?	N
83.	The naked human body is a pleasing sight.	Y	?	N
84.	It would not disturb me over much if my sex partner had sexual relations with someone else, as long as he returned to me.	Y	?	N
85.	Some forms of love-making are disgusting to me.	Y	?	N

Please underline the correct answer

86. If you were invited to see a 'blue' film would you:
(a) Accept   (b) Refuse

87. If you were offered a highly pornographic book, would you:
(a) Accept it   (b) Reject it

88. If you were invited to take part in an orgy, would you:
     (a) Take part   (b) Refuse

89. Have you ever suffered from impotence:
     (a) Never   (d) Often
     (b) Once or twice   (e) More often than not
     (c) Several times   (f) Always

90. Rate the strength of the influences that inhibit you sexually
     (moral, aesthetic, religious, ets.) from 10 (terribly strong,
     completely inhibiting) to 1 (very weak and almost non-existent).

     Rating:

Bibliography

Ader, R. (1981). *Psychoneuroimmunology.* New York: Academic Press.

Ader, R., and Cohen, N. (1981). Conditioned immunopharmacologic response. In: Ader, R. (ed.), *Psychoneuroimmunology* 281–319. New York: Academic Press.

Altman, D. (1971). *Homosexual Oppression and Liberation.* New York: Avon.

Altman, D. (1982). *The Homosexualization of America.* Boston: Beacon Press.

Andrew, G. M., and Ross, M. W. (1981). A short form of the Bem Sex Role Inventory. *Journal of Psychiatric Treatment and Evaluation* 3:563–66.

Armytage, W. H. G. (1980). Changing incidence and patterns of sexually transmitted diseases. *Proceedings of the 15th Annual Symposium of the Eugenics Society* 15:159–70.

Arya, O. P., and Bennett, F. J. (1967). Venereal disease in an elite group (university students) in East Africa. *British Journal of Venereal Diseases* 43:275–79.

Austin, D. F. (1982). Etiological clues from descriptive epidemiology: Squamous carcinoma of the rectum or anus. *National Cancer Institute Monographs* 62:89–90.

Bell, A. P., and Weinberg, M. S. (1978). *Homosexualities: A Study of Diveristy Among Men and Women.* Melbourne: Macmillan.

Bem, S. L. (1974). The measurement of psychological androgyny. *Journal of Consulting and Clinical Psychology* 42:155–62.

Bhanji, S., and Mahony, J. H. D. (1978). The value of a psychiatric service within the venereal disease clinic. *British Journal of Venereal Diseases* 54:266–68.

Blalock, J. E. (1984). The immune system as a senory organ. *Journal of Immunology* 132:1067–70.

Bolling, D. R. (1977). Prevalence, goals and complications of heterosexual anal intercourse in a gynaecologic population. *Journal of Reproductive Medicine* 19:120–24.

Burns, C. R. (1974). Diseases versus healths: Some legacies in the philosophies of modern medical science.

In: Engelhardt, H. T., and Spicker, S. F. (eds.), *Evaluation and Explanation in the Medical Sciences,* 29–47. Dordrecht: D. Reidel.

Burrell, C. J., Cameron, A. S., Hart, G., Melbourne, J., and Beal, R. W. (1983). Hepatitis B reservoirs and attack rates in an Australian community: A basis for vaccination and crossinfection policies. *Medical Journal of Australia 2*:492–96.

Butler, S. (1872/1935). *Erewhon, or: Over the Range.* Harmondsworth, Middlesex: Penguin.

Canton, G., Santonastaso, P., and Fraccon, I. G. (1984). Life events, abnormal illness behavior, and appendectomy. *General Hospital Psychiatry 6*:191–95.

Cass, V. C. (1979). Homosexual identity formation: A theoretical model. *Journal of Homosexuality 4*:219–35.

Catalan, J., Bradley, M., Gallwey, J., and Hawton, K. (1981). Sexual dysfunction and psychiatric morbidity in patients attending a clinic for sexually transmitted diseases. *British Journal of Psychiatry 138*:292–96.

Christenson, B., Brostrom, C., Bottinger, M., Hermanson, J., Welland, O., Ryd, G., Berg, J. V. R., and Sjoblom, R. (1982). An epidemic outbreak of hepatitis A among homosexual men in Stockholm. *American Journal of Epidemiology 116*:599–607.

Clayer, J. R., Bookless, C., and Ross, M. W. (1984). Neurosis and conscious symptom exaggeration: Its differentiation by the Illness Behavior Questionnaire. *Journal of Psychosomatic Research 28*:237–41.

Comaroff, J. (1982). Medicine: Symbol and ideology. In: Wright, P., and Treacher, A. (eds.), *The Problem of Medical Knowledge: Examining the Social Construction of Medicine,* 49–68. Edinburgh: Edinburgh University Press.

Daling, J. R., Weiss, N. S., Klopfenstein, L. L., Cochran, L. E., Chow, W. H., and Daifuku, R. (1982). Correlates of homosexual behavior and the incidence of anal cancer. *Journal of the American Medical Association 247*:1988–90.

Dardick, L., and Grady, K. (1980). Openness between gay persons and health professionals. *Annals of Internal Medicine 93*:115–19.

Darrow, W. W. (1981). Social and psychologic aspects of the sexually transmitted diseases: A different view. *Cutis 27*:307–20.

Darrow, W. W., Barrett, D., Jay, K., and Young, A. (1981). The gay report on sexually transmitted diseases. *American Journal of Public Health 71*:1004–11.

Eysenck, H. J. (1976). *Sex and Personality.* London:

Abacus.

Eysenck, H. J., and Eysenck, S. (1975). *Manual of the Eysenck Personality Questionnaire.* London: University of London Press.

Fleck, L. (1935). *The Genesis and Development of a Scientific Fact.* Bradley, F., and Trenn, T. J. (transls.) (1979). Chicago: University of Chicago Press.

Fluker, J. L. (1981). Homosexuality and sexually transmitted diseases. *British Journal of Hospital Medicine 26:* 265–69.

Fluker, J. L. (1983). The perils of promiscuity. *Journal of Psychosomatic Research 27:*153–56.

Freedman, M. (1971). *Homosexuality and Psychological Functioning.* Belmont, California: Brooks-Cole.

Fulford, K. W. M., Catterall, R. D., Hoinville, E., Lim, K. S., and Wilson, G. D. (1983a). Social and psychological factors in the distribution of STD in male clinic attenders. I. Demographic and social factors. *British Journal of Venereal Diseases 59:*376–80.

Fulford, K. W. M., Catterall, R. D., Hoinville, E., Lim, K. S., and Wilson, G. D. (1983b). Social and psychological factors in the distribution of STD in male clinic attenders. II. Personality disorders, psychiatric illness, and abnormal sexual attitudes. *British Journal of Venereal Diseases 59:*381–85.

Fulford, K. W. M., Catterall, R. D., Hoinville, E., Lim, K. S., and Wilson, G. D. (1983c). Social and psychological factors in the distribution of STD male clinic attenders. III. Sexual activity. *British Journal of Venereal Diseases 59:*386–93.

Gebhard, P. H., and Johnson, A. B. (1979). *The Kinsey Data: Marginal Tabulations of the 1938–1963 Interviews Conducted by the Institute for Sex Research.* Philadelphia: W. B. Saunders.

Goode, E., and Troiden, R. R. (1980). Correlates and accompaniments of promiscuous sex among male homosexuals. *Psychiatry 43:*51–59.

Greene, W. A., Betts, R. F., Ochitill, H. N., Iker, H. P., and Douglas, R. G. (1978). Psychosocial factors and immunity: Preliminary report. *Psychosomatic Medicine 40:*87.

Groddeck, G. (1929). *The Unknown Self: A New Psychological Approach to the Problems of Life, with Special Reference to Disease.* London: C. W. Daniel.

Haist, M., and Hewitt, J. (1974). The butch-fem dichotomy in male homosexual behavior. *Journal of Sex Research 10:*68–75.

Handsfield, H. H. (1981). Sexually transmitted diseases in homosexual men. *American Journal of Public Health* 71:989–90.

Hart, G. (1973a). Social aspects of venereal disease. I. Sociological determinants of venereal disease. *British Journal of Venereal Diseases* 49:542–47.

Hart, G. (1973b). Social aspects of venereal disease. II. Relationship of personality to other sociological determinants of venereal disease. *British Journal of Venereal Diseases* 49:548–52.

Hart, G. (1973c). Psychological aspects of venereal disease in a war environment. *Social Science and Medicine* 7:455–67.

Hart, G. (1974a). Factors influencing venereal infection in a war environment. *British Journal of Venereal Diseases* 50:68–72.

Hart, G. (1974b). Social and psychological aspects of venereal disease in Papua New Guinea. *British Journal of Venereal Diseases* 50:453–58.

Hart, G. (1975). Sexual behavior in a war environment. *Journal of Sex Research* 11:218–26.

Hart, G. (1977). *Sexual Maladjustment and Disease: An Introduction to Modern Venereology.* Chicago: Nelson-Hall.

Henderson, R. (1977). Improving sexually transmitted disease health services for gays: A national perspective. *Sexually Transmitted Diseases* 4:58–62.

Hooker, E. (1964). Male homosexual life styles and venereal disease. *Proceedings of the World Forum on Syphilis and Other Treponematoses.* Public Health Service Publication 997. Washington, DC: U.S. Government Printing Office.

Hooker, E. (1965). An empirical study of some relations between sexual patterns and gender identity in male homosexuals. In: Money, J. (ed.), *Sex Research: New Developments,* 24–52. New York: Holt, Rinehart & Winston.

Humphreys, R. A. L. (1970). *Tearoom Trade: A Study of Impersonal Sex in Public Places.* London: Duckworth.

Israel, J. (1972). Stipulations and construction in the social sciences. In: Israel, J., and Tajfel, H. (eds), *The Context of Social Psychology: A Critical Assessment.* London: Academic Press.

Jemmott, J. B., and Locke, S. E. (1984). Psychosocial factors, immunologic mediation, and human susceptibility to infectious diseases: How much do we know? *Psychological Bulletin* 95:78–108.

Jenkins, C. D., Rosenman, R. H., and Friedman, M.

(1967). Development of an objective test for the determination of the coronary-prone behavior pattern in
employed men. *Journal of Chronic Diseases 20*:371–79.

Judson, F. N. (1977). Sexually transmitted diseases in
homosexual men. *Sexually Transmitted Diseases*
4:76–78.

Locke, S. E., and Heisel, S. J. (1977). The influence of
stress and emotions on the human immune response.
Biofeedback and Self-Regulation 2:320.

Locke, S. E., Hurst, M. W., Heisel, F. J., Kraus, L., and
Williams, M. (1979). The influence of stress and other
psychological factors on human immunity. Paper presented at the 36th Annual Meeting of the Psychosomatic
Society, Dallas, Texas, March.

Kelus, J. (1973). Social and behavioural aspects of venereal disease. *British Journal of Venereal Diseases*
49:167–70.

Kinsey, A. C., Pomeroy, W. B., and Martin, C. E. (1948).
Sexual Behavior in the Human Male. Philadelphia:
W. B. Saunders.

Krafft-Ebing, R. von (1886). *Psychopathia Sexualis.*
Wedeck, H. E. (transl.) (1965). New York: G. P.
Putnam's.

Kuhn, T. S. (1970). *The Structure of Scientific Revolu-
tions* (2d ed.). Chicago: University of Chicago Press.

McDonald, A. P. (1974). Identification and measurement of
multidimensional attitudes toward equality of the sexes.
Journal of Homosexuality 1:165–82.

McGreil, M. (1977). *Prejudice and Tolerance in Ireland.*
Dublin: College of Industrial Relations.

McMillan, A., and Lee, F. D. (1981). Sigmoidoscopic and
microscopic appearance of the rectal mucosa in homosexual men. *Gut 22*:1035–41.

McNair, D. M., Lorr, M., and Droppleman, L. F. (1971).
Manual for the Profile of Mood States. San Diego:
Educational and Industrial Testing Service.

Monjan, A. A. (1981). Stress and immunologic competence:
Studies in animals. In: Ader, R. (ed.), *Psychoneuroimmunology,* 185–228. New York: Academic Press.

Morton, R. S. (1966). *Venereal Diseases.* Harmondsworth,
Middlesex: Penguin.

Nicol, C. S. (1963). Venereal diseases, moral standards
and public opinion. *British Journal of Venereal Diseases 39*:168–72.

Ostrow, D. G. (1984). Psychovenereology: A new direction
for the 1980s or a throwback to the 1950s? *Sexually
Transmitted Diseases 11*:182.

Ostrow, D. G., and Altman, N. L. (1983). Sexually transmitted diseases and homosexuality. *Sexually Trans-mitted Diseases 10*:208–15.

Oriel, J. D. (1971). Anal warts and anal coitus. *British Journal of Venereal Diseases 47*:373.

Oriel, J. D. (1982). The global pattern of sexually transmitted diseases. *South African Medical Journal 61*:993–98.

Palmblad, J. (1981). Stress and immunologic competence: Studies in man. In: Ader, R. (ed.), *Psychoneuroimmunology,* 229–57. New York: Academic Press.

Pankhurst, C. (1913). *The Great Scourge and How To End It.* London: E. Pankhurst.

Parkin, A. (1981). The Dunstan governments: A political synopsis. In: Parkin, A., and Patience, A. (eds.), *The Dunstan Decade: Social Democracy at the State Level,* 1–21. Melbourne: Longman Cheshire.

Pauly, I. B., and Goldstein, S. (1970). Physicians' attitudes in treating homosexuals. *Medical Aspects of Human Sexuality 4*:26–45.

Pedder, J. R., and Goldberg, D. P. (1970). A survey by questionnaire of psychiatric disturbance in patients attending a venereal disease clinic. *British Journal of Venereal Diseases 46*:58–61.

Perris, C., Jacobsson, L., Lindstrom, H., von Knorring, L., and Perris, H. (1980). Development of a new inventory for assessing memories of parental rearing behavior. *Acta Psychiatrica Scandinavica 61*:265–74.

Pilowsky, I. (1969). Abnormal illness behaviour. *British Journal of Medical Psychology 42*:347–51.

Pilowsky, I. (1978). A general classification of abnormal illness behaviour. *British Journal of Medical Psychology 51*:131–37.

Pilowsky, I., and Spence, N. D. (1983). *Manual for the Illness Behaviour Questionnaire* (2d ed.) Adelaide: Department of Psychiatry, University of Adelaide.

Rechy, J. (1963). *City of Night.* London: Panther.

Riess, A. J. (1961). The social integration of peers and queers. *Social Problems 9*:102–20.

Robertson, P., and Schacter, J. (1981). Failure to identify venereal disease in a lesbian population. *Sexually Transmitted Diseases 8*:75–76.

Rose, R. M. (1980). Endocrine responses to stressful psychological events. *Psychiatric Clinics of North America 3*:251–76.

Rosebury, T. (1972). *Microbes and Morals: The Strange Story of Venereal Disease.* London: Secker and Warburg.

Rosenberg, M. (1965). *Society and the Adolescent Self-*

Image. Princeton: Princeton University Press.

Ross, M. W. (1978). The relationship of perceived societal hostility, conformity, and psychological adjustment in homosexual males. *Journal of Homosexuality* 4:157–68.

Ross, M. W. (1979). Homosexuality and venereal disease. *British Journal of Sexual Medicine* 6(46):32–33.

Ross, M. W. (1981). Attitudes of male homosexuals to venereal disease clinics. *Medical Journal of Australia* 2:670–71.

Ross, M. W. (1982). Social factors in homosexually acquired venereal disease: A comparison between Sweden and Australia. *British Journal of Venereal Diseases* 58:263–68.

Ross, M. W. (1983). *The Married Homosexual Man: A Psychological Study.* London: Routledge and Kegan Paul.

Ross, M. W. (1984a). Sexually transmitted diseases in homosexual men: A study of four societies. *British Journal of Venereal Diseases* 60:52–55.

Ross, M. W. (1984b). Sociological and psychological predictors of STD infection in homosexual men: A study of four countries. *British Journal of Venereal Diseases* 60:110–13.

Ross, M. W. (1984c). Psychovenereology and acquired immune deficiency syndrome. In: Nichols, S. E., and Ostrow, D. G. (eds.), *Psychiatric Implications of Acquired Immune Deficiency Syndrome,* 111–21. Washington, DC: American Psychiatric Association Press.

Ross, M. W. (1984d). Predictors of partner numbers in homosexual men: Psychosocial factors in four societies. *Sexually Transmitted Diseases* 11:119–22.

Ross, M. W. (1985a). Sexual practices as risk factors for sexually transmitted diseases in homosexual men. *European Journal of Sexually Transmitted Diseases* 2:159–62.

Ross, M. W. (1985b). Psychosocial factors in admitting to homosexuality in sexually transmitted disease clinics. *Sexually Transmitted Diseases* 12:83–86.

Ross, M. W. (1985c). Illness behavior in sexually transmitted disease clinic attenders. *Sexually Transmitted Diseases,* in press.

Ross, M. W. (1985d). Partner preference characteristics in homosexual men: A comparison of four societies. Submitted for publication.

Ross, M. W. (1985e). Actual and anticipated societal reaction to homosexuality and adjustment in two societies. *Journal of Sex Research* 21:40–55.

Ross, M. W., Campbell, R. L., and Clayer, J. R. (1982).

New inventory for measurement of parental rearing patterns: An English form of the EMBU. *Acta Psychiatrica Scandinavica 66*:499–507.

Ross, M. W., Clayer, J. R., and Campbell, R. L. (1983). Dimensions of child-rearing practices: Factor structure of the EMBU. *Acta Psychiatrica Scandinavica 68*:476–83.

Ross, M. W., Rogers, L. J., and McCulloch, H. (1978). Stigma, sex and society: A new look at gender differentiation and sexual variation. *Journal of Homosexuality 3*:315–30.

Ross, M. W., and Stalstrom, O. W. (1984). Attitudes to venereal disease clinics in Finnish homosexual men. *European Journal of Sexually Transmitted Diseases 1*:169–71.

Ross, M. W., and Talikka, A. (1978). Finland and homosexuality. *Psychiatric News 13*(14):2, 10.

Sandholzer, T. Z. (1980). Physician attitudes and other factors affecting the incidence of sexually transmitted diseases in homosexual males. *Journal of Homosexuality 5*:325–28.

Schofield, M. (1976). *Promiscuity*. London: Victor Gollancz.

Schreeder, M. T., Thompson, S. E., Hadler, S. C., Berquist, K. R., Zaidi, A., Maynard, J. E., Ostrow, D., Judson, F. N., Braff, E. H., Nylund, T., Moore, J. N., Gardner, P., Doto, I. L., and Reynolds, G. (1982). Hepatitis B in homosexual men: Prevalence of infection and factors related to transmission. *Journal of Infectious Diseases 146*:7–15.

Stamm, W. E., Koutsky, L. A., Benedetti, J. K., Jourden, J. L., Brunham, R. C., and Holmes, K. K. (1984). *Chlamydia trachomatis* urethral infections in men: Prevalence, risk factors, and clinical manifestations. *Annals of Internal Medicine 100*:47–51.

Suhonen, R., Wallenius, J., Haukka, K., Elo, O., and Lassus, A. (1976). Syphilis, homosexuality and legislation. *Dermatologica 152*:363–66.

Thin, R. N., and Smith, D. M. (1976). Some characteristics of homosexual men. *British Journal of Venereal Diseases 52*:161–64.

Truax, C. B., and Carkhuff, R. R. (1967). *Toward Effective Counselling and Psychotherapy: Training and Practice*. Chicago: Aldine.

Waugh, M. A. (1972). Studies in the recent epidemiology of early syphilis in West London. *British Journal of Venereal Diseases 48*:534.

Weinberg, M. S., and Williams, C. J. (1974). *Male Homo-*

sexuals: Their Problems and Adaptations. New York: Oxford University Press.

Wells, B. W. P. (1969). Personality characteristics of VD patients. *British Journal of Social and Clinical Psychology* 8:246–52.

Wells, B. W. P., and Schofield, C. B. S. (1972). Personality characteristics of homosexual men suffering from sexually transmitted diseases. *British Journal of Venereal Diseases* 48:75–78.

West, D. J. (1977). *Homosexuality Re-examined.* London: Duckworth.

Wilcox, R. R. (1973). Homosexuality and venereal disease in the United Kingdom. *British Journal of Venereal Diseases* 49:329–34.

Wild, R. A. (1978). *Social Stratification in Australia.* Sydney: George Allen and Unwin.

World Health Organization (1975). Social and health aspects of sexually transmitted diseases. *Public Health Papers* 65. Geneva: WHO.

Index

About the Author

Dr. Michael Ross is AIDS Coordinator of the South Australian Health Commission, and Senior Lecturer in Psychiatry and Community Medicine at the Flinders University Medical School in Adelaide, Australia. Born in New Zealand, he studied at the Universities of Wellington and New York, completed his doctoral research at the Universities of Melbourne and Stockholm, and his postdoctoral work at the University of Helsinki. In 1980 he was awarded the Hugo G. Beigel Prize of the Society for the Scientific Study of Sex for his research on male homosexuality, and is a member of the editorial board of the *Journal of Homosexuality*. To date he has published nearly a hundred scientific papers and chapters in the areas of sexuality, psychiatry, and sexually transmitted diseases, and three books: *The Married Homosexual Man: A Psychological Study; Homosexuality and Social Sex Roles;* and with William A. W. Walters, *Transsexualism*.